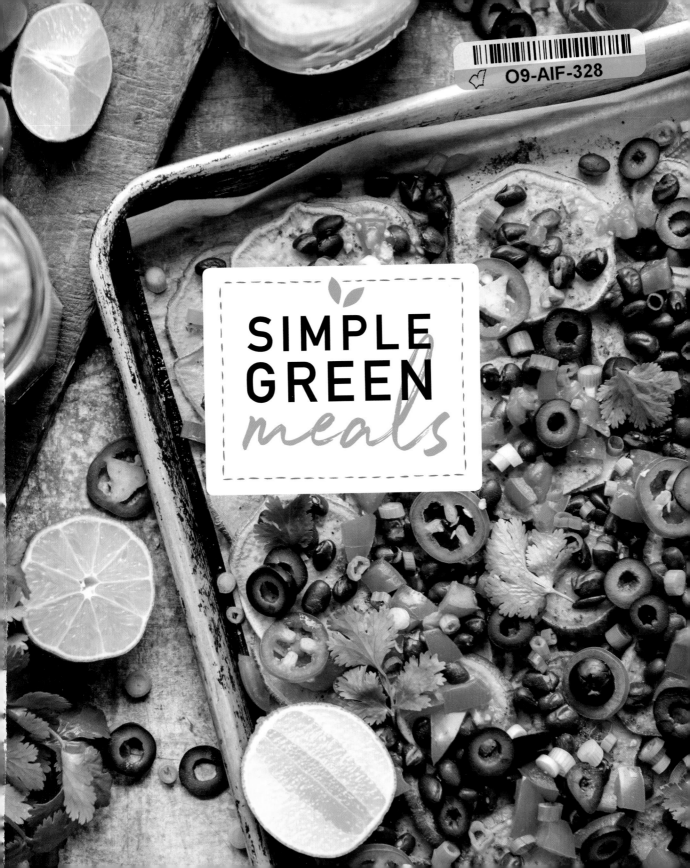

SIMPLE
GREEN
meals

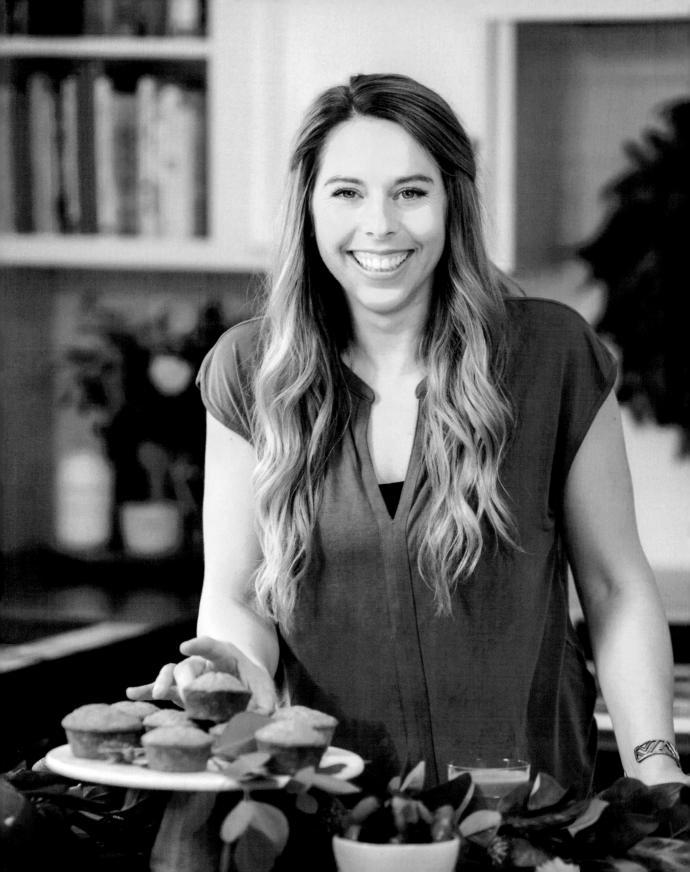

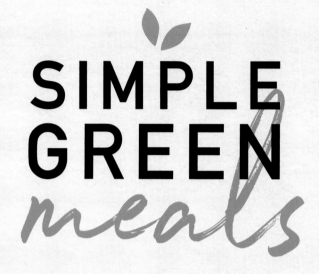

SIMPLE
GREEN
meals

100+ plant-powered recipes
to thrive from the inside out

Jen Hansard

with Lindsey Johnson

RODALE

Copyright © 2018 by Jen Hansard

All rights reserved.
Published in the United States by Rodale Books,
an imprint of the Crown Publishing Group, a division
of Penguin Random House LLC, New York.
crownpublishing.com
rodalebooks.com

RODALE and the Plant colophon are registered
trademarks of Penguin Random House LLC.

Library of Congress Cataloging-in-Publication Data is available.

ISBN 978-1-63565-009-9
Ebook ISBN 978-1-63565-010-5

Printed in the United States of America

Cover and book design by Nicole LaRoche
Cover and food photographs by Lindsey Rose Johnson
Lifestyle photographs by Jim and Ilde Cook of Cookhouse Media
Pages 2 and 11 photographs by Liz and Ryan Bower
Page 7 photograph by Daniel Mottayaw

10 9 8 7 6 5 4

First Edition

To community—no matter where we go,

may we continue to find one another

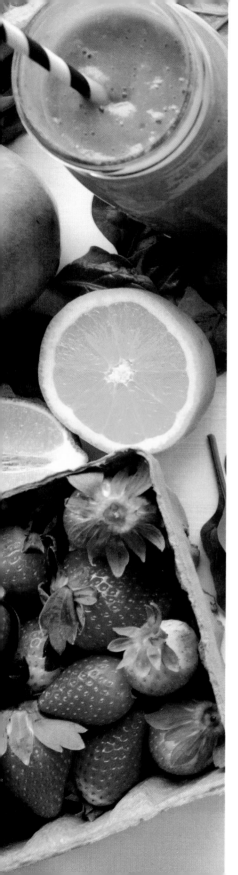

CONTENTS

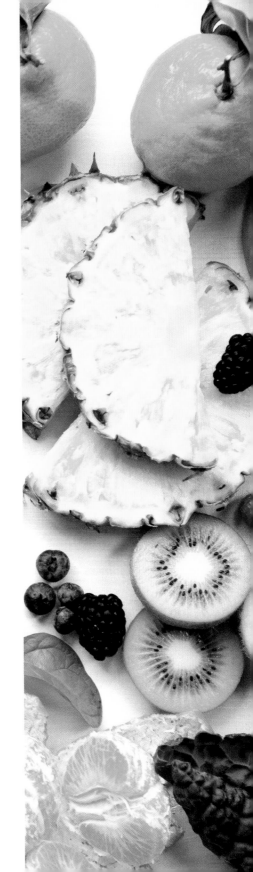

part two
PLANT-POWERED RECIPES

part three
HELPFUL RESOURCES

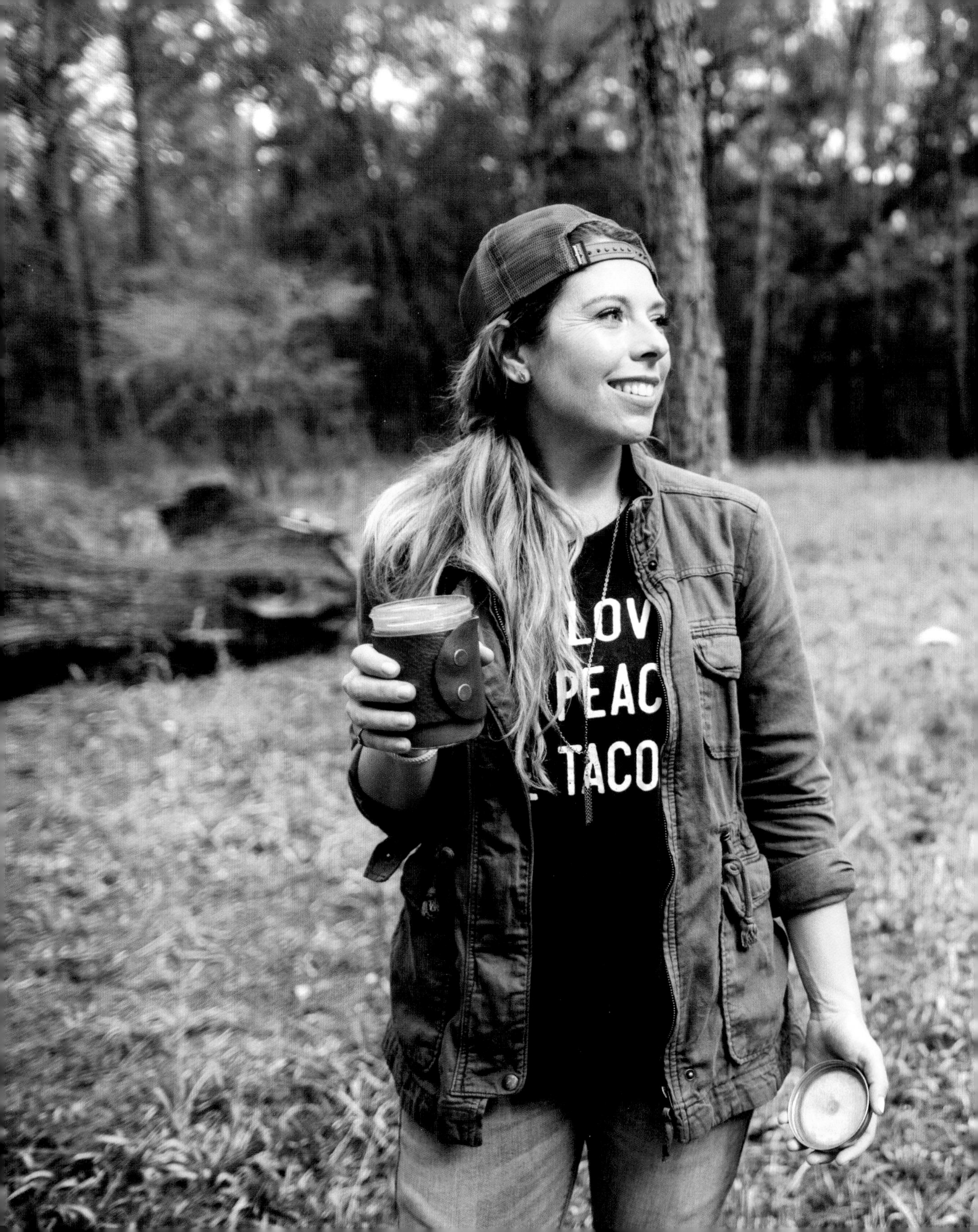
LOV
PEAC
TACO

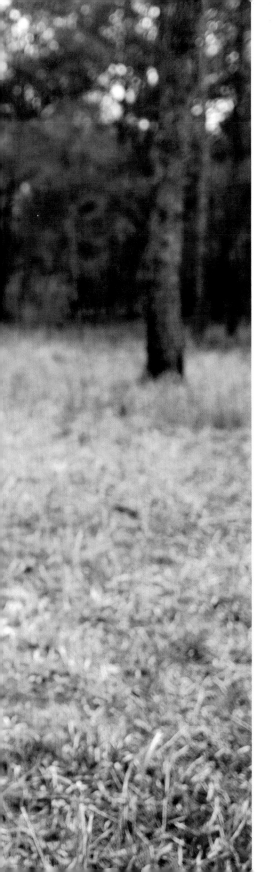

INTRODUCTION

I remember the night my husband, Ryan, asked me a simple (but loaded) question. We had just finished dinner and gotten the kids to bed. I was feeling run down from another day of cramming what felt like a week's worth of activities, appointments, and errands into a single day. We were in the kitchen putting the dishes away, and Ryan was talking about the next hobby he'd like to get into—he was thinking of transitioning from juggling into sculpting papier-mâché animals. It was a fun idea, and I was sort of listening, but I was mainly thinking about how good the bed was going to feel in 15 more minutes. I was exhausted. Then he asked me this:

"What do you love to do, Jen?"

My mind went blank. I couldn't think of anything. I couldn't fathom adding something else into my life—let alone something fun—because there was so much that I felt like I *had* to do. I was barely keeping my head above water, allowing everyone and everything in my life to become a priority and pushing my needs further and further down. Instead of putting on my oxygen mask first in an emergency so I could help others, I was giving it right away to someone else and forgoing my own. The more I did for others before my own needs, the less I recognized myself. The little flame flickering deep inside me was getting smaller and smaller. If anything else was added to my crazy-packed life, I was scared the flame might blow out.

Yet Ryan's question stuck with me, and I couldn't shake it. Why couldn't I think of something that I wanted to do just for myself? Heck, I was the girl who jumped into the snowmelt river with my high school running buddies after a 4-mile trail run in the High Sierras. In college, I juggled three jobs, married my high school sweetheart, got pregnant, and then graduated with two degrees—in that order. I did it all because I loved it all and wanted it all. I didn't make excuses . . . I made ways.

Where was that Jen now, and who was standing in that kitchen putting away the dishes like a zombie?

Ryan's question was the wake-up call I needed, the signal to burn a little brighter and live as a truer, more passionate version of myself. I set off on my own adventure: a wellness adventure.

FOOD IS THY MEDICINE

My life didn't change all at once after that, but it took a sharp turn with a chiropractor (known to my friends as my "hippy doctor"). After adjusting my back, he'd spend time explaining the problems with the American food system. He used terms I'd never heard before, like *trace minerals* and *gut health*, and he got me watching food documentaries. Pretty quickly, our family gave up corn syrup, food dyes, and most dairy products because of him. We avoided the main food distributors that used cheap, harmful ingredients and invested our small amount of money into brands we could believe in that made quality ingredients.

Then we began drinking green smoothies, which boosted our energy levels and immune systems. My excitement led to starting the company Simple Green Smoothies with my friend Jadah Sellner, who was my partner in kale for 5 years. As I drank more green smoothies, I started craving more plants. I literally would happily choose a side salad over french fries at a restaurant. Who was I?! I splurged on 15 cookbooks and started preparing meals that celebrated plants. A vegetarian since I was 16 years old, it's pretty comical that it wasn't until I turned 28 that I actually started *eating* vegetables. Until then, grilled cheese, Lucky Charms, and bean burritos were my jam.

I knew that if I wanted this new way of living to stick, I needed to invite others along for the journey. I made friends with a fellow foodie named Lindsey Johnson, and she started cocreating plant-based recipes at Simple Green Smoothies. Her enthusiasm for flavors and variety was contagious, and I couldn't get enough of it. She's been our rawkstar recipe creator ever since. Her passion and talent are infused throughout this book. If you fall in love with a recipe, it's because Lindsey added her magical touch and made it look so pretty.

Eating more plants gave me the energy I needed to go after the things I wanted most. Sure, I still had a lot on my plate, because what woman doesn't? Yet I decided it was okay to move myself up on the list of to-dos and add more *me* to my life. It was time to figure out "what I love to do" and go after it. This book is in celebration of that.

Since that night in the kitchen, I've flown planes, jumped off cliffs, snorkeled in national parks, helped build a library in Guatemala, and run a 100-K ultramarathon trail run that lasted 18 hours. Food gave me the energy to take that next step and dive deeper into what I am here on this beautiful planet to do. I've transformed from exhausted and burnt out to energetic and passionate. And I know the same can happen for you! Cooking and eating nutrient-dense, whole foods to nourish your body will help you answer this question as authentic as ever: *What do you love to do?*

Peace, love, and leafy greens,
Jen Hansard

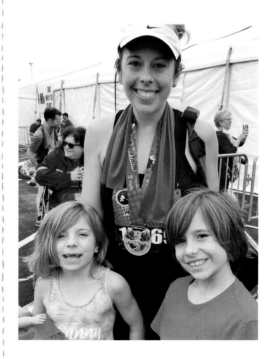

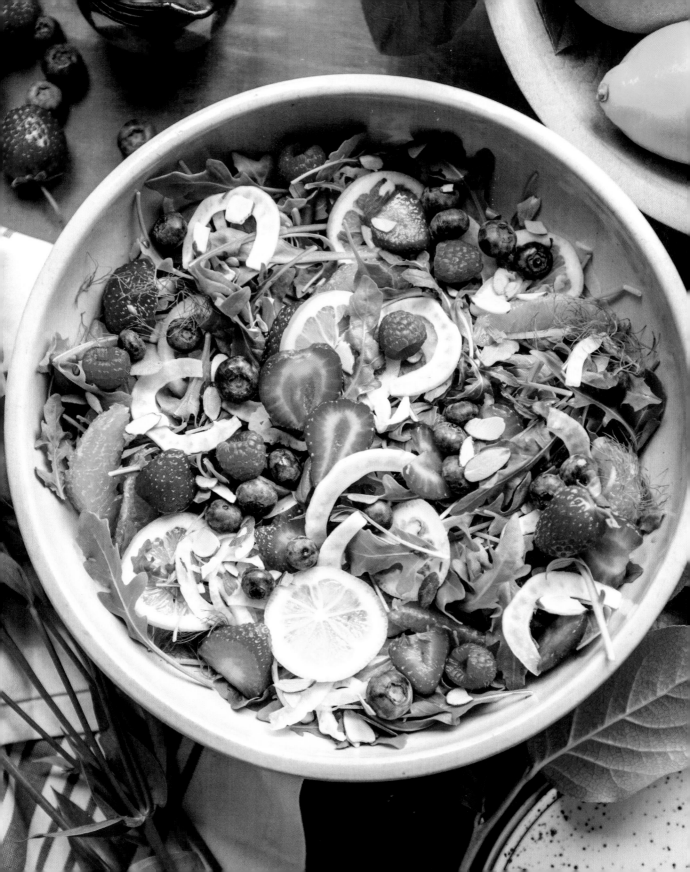

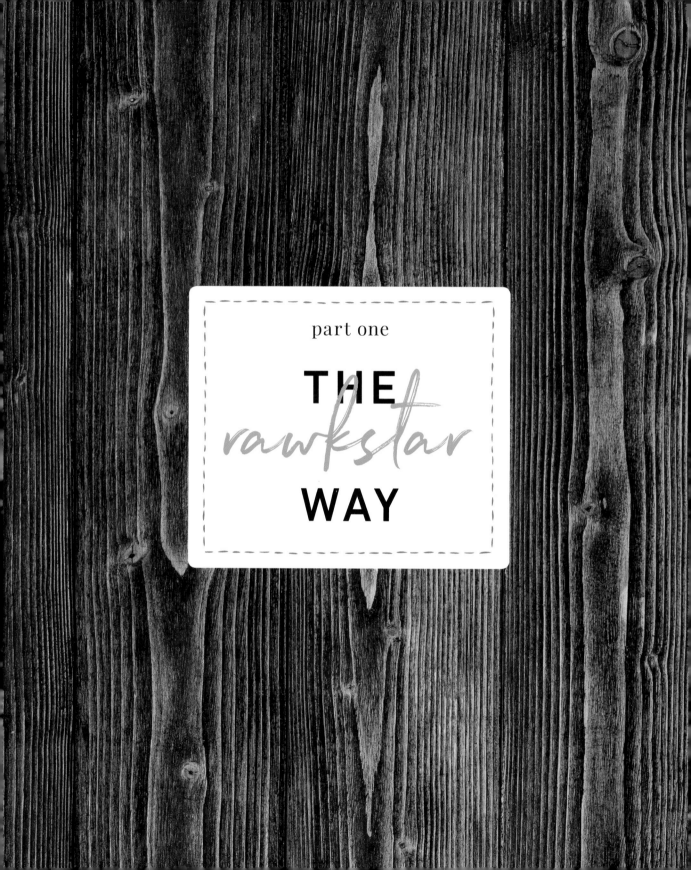

part one

THE
rawkstar
WAY

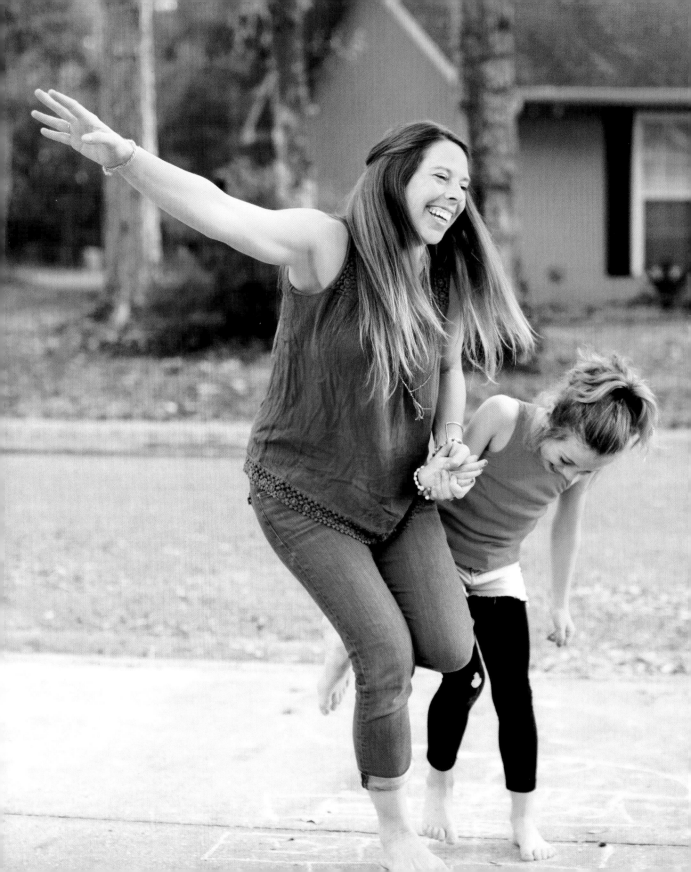

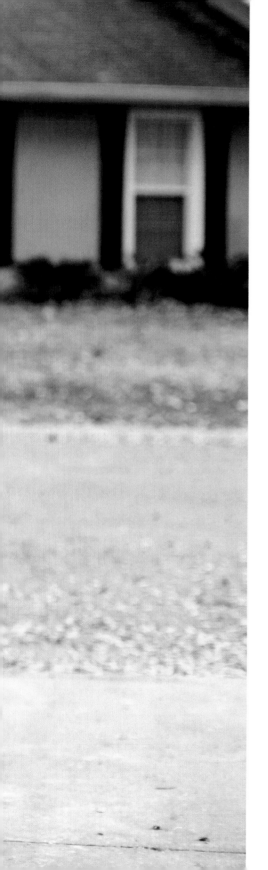

PLANT-POWERED
passion
fuel your body,
live out your passion

This book is not just a recipe book. Sure, it has 100 amazing recipes that will help you feel your best, but I would be doing you a disservice if it was just that. The thing is, once you start eating plant-powered foods that replenish your energy levels and nourish your body, the obstacles that were holding you back are gone—you're ready to take on the world. We're gonna make health *and* passion key pieces to who you are every single day and leave exhaustion and uncertainty in the dust.

So let's discover your passion!

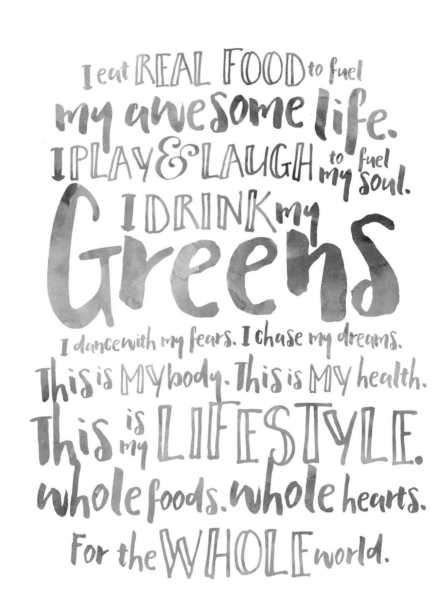

I eat REAL FOOD to fuel my awesome life. I PLAY & LAUGH to fuel my soul. I DRINK my Greens I dance with my fears. I chase my dreams. This is MY body. This is MY health. This is my LIFESTYLE. whole foods. whole hearts. For the WHOLE world.

— THE RAWKSTAR MANIFESTO —

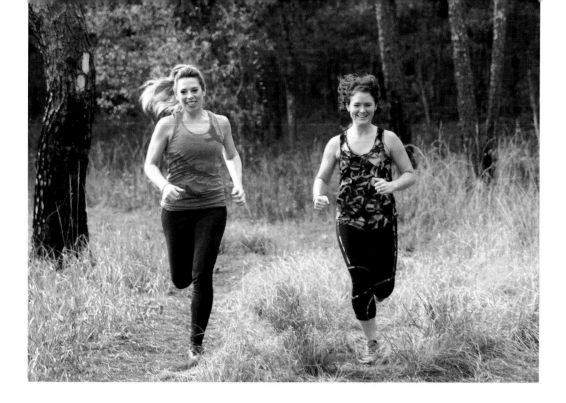

DISCOVERING MY PASSIONS

I'm often asked what made me want to run ultramarathons or take flying lessons. The truth is, I've always been drawn to those things—always had a place carved out for them in my heart—but there was a time when I just didn't realize it, because I was so tired and stressed in my day-to-day life. I had tucked those dreams so deep inside of me that I forgot they were there!

In 2011, I had begun taking my *physical* health seriously by focusing on improved nutrition through green smoothies and whole foods. Yet it wasn't until 2015 that I started taking my

mental health seriously. I hired a life coach, and together we set off on a journey toward my best self. She helped me unpack the desires of my heart and go after them. I read books like *Essentialism* by Greg McKeown and *Rising Strong* by Brené Brown. I soon found myself scheduling time for *me*. It was as if I had been holding my breath for years, and now I could finally exhale. It felt amazing. I began running in the morning. I scheduled my runs into my calendar, and so I honored them. I've always loved moving my body and pushing its limits. The days I ran seemed to be the best days in my week: I was more productive at work, my relationships were stronger, and I was eating better. So, like Forrest Gump, I just kept running. Through this simple routine, I was unleashing the bold, daring woman I was created to be.

I had hit a major milestone in my company, Simple Green Smoothies, and was in awe of how connected I felt with my kids and husband. I was so happy and proud of how far I had come. Then my coach asked me a question.

"How are you going to celebrate?"

Well, I honestly hadn't thought of that. To me, celebrating was the moment of acknowledgment after completing a blog post, or sleeping soundly after a long day of juggling work and taking the kids to baseball and gymnastics. So I tried to find a more meaningful way to celebrate my accomplishments. *I could go out to dinner with Ryan, or head to Target and get a new outfit and some new home decor,* I thought, but I knew those answers weren't quite there. So I kept digging and eventually blurted out, "I could fly a plane!" Yep, that's the one that made my heart skip a beat.

That was how I would celebrate my transition from being overwhelmed and exhausted to thriving and passionate.

On my 33rd birthday, I got in that plane and soared through the sky with my instructor, staring down at the beautiful world from 10,000 feet up.

The funny thing about dreams is that when you bring them to life, they are often bigger than you had hoped. As the tires touched down on the landing strip, I knew that I would be flying a plane myself one day. Five months later, my instructor handed the controls fully over to me for our flight: I was in charge of takeoff, flying over my house, and landing. It wasn't the smoothest flight, but I was a pilot that day.

Having people in your corner who can ask the tough questions, push you toward dreams, and stand by your side as you go after them will make all the difference. Take a minute and think of who those people are in your life. Whom do you open up to? Who supports you? Thank them for being there for you in that special way. I am so thankful for my husband, who asked me the tough question—"What do you love to do, Jen?"—that tired night in the kitchen, and for my coach for helping me find the answer and go for it. Who is there for you? If someone doesn't immediately come to mind, consider who in your life could fill that role. You need someone in your corner encouraging you to go after the things that matter most to *you*.

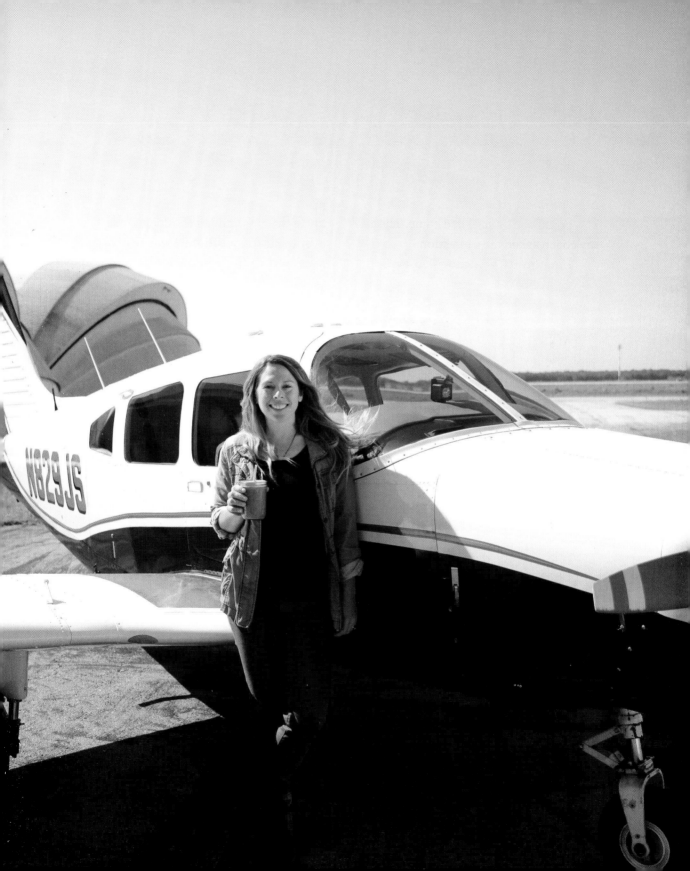

PASSIONATE PEOPLE YOU SHOULD KNOW

One of the greatest blessings of my job is meeting incredible people who become my friends. I asked a few to share their passions to help you see how unique this can look for each of us.

WHITNEY ENGLISH, *homeschool mom and founder of the Day Designer*

@whitneyenglish

I'm currently pursuing a passion for textiles and interiors. My husband is a real estate agent here in Oklahoma, and we are both passionate about helping people build a home here.

CHELSEA DINSMORE, *chief inspiration officer of Live Your Legend*

@chelseadinsmore

I have a big passion for travel and have a small side project to educate people about how I have traveled the globe for the past 7 years, spending almost nothing on airline flights. I am also incredibly passionate about nourishing the mind, body, and spirit.

LINDSAY OSTROM, *blogger at Pinch of Yum*

@pinchofyum

My passion is for practicality. We all have an abundance of beautiful ideas at our fingertips on Pinterest and Instagram, but ironically, those perfect grids often make us feel less-than about our lives instead of awesome and empowered. As a food blogger, I love to give people a recipe they will actually make—not too intimidating, but just exciting enough to make them feel capable and creative.

AMY PORTERFIELD, *mom, wife, online marketing expert and educator, and host of the top-ranked podcast, Online Marketing Made Easy*

@amyporterfield

My passion is to help my students break away from the 9-to-5 jobs they hate and into building online businesses they absolutely love. I love to see the "lightbulb moments" when something clicks and things start to fall into place. It's pretty special to witness!

STEVE KAMB, *founder and rebel leader of NerdFitness.com*

@nerdfitness

I have a passion for learning! I read two books per week to keep my mind sharp (putting the "nerd" in Nerd Fitness!). I'm currently taking violin lessons and always trying to develop a new fitness skill, too (currently planches and handstands).

ASHLEY AND GRAHAM SCOBEY, *high school sweethearts turned wedding photography team at Scobey Photography*

@thescobeys

As a whole, our greatest passion is adventure and living life with our whole hearts. Homeschooling our kiddos and traveling are two really big parts of that for us right now. We love getting to spend time together, take risks, and try new things.

find your passion worksheet

This worksheet will help you dig deep to figure out what lights you up and how you can fuel your passion. My coach, Christen Bavero of ThinkHuman, created it just for you. I can't wait to hear where it takes you! Share on social media and tag me @simplegreensmoothies so I can celebrate with you, okay?

1. What is important to you, or what really matters to you? List as many as you can.

_____

_____

_____

_____

_____

_____

_____

_____

2. What things fuel you but are not currently in your life? List as many as you can.

_____

_____

_____

_____

_____

_____

_____

3. Focus on one thing you wrote down in question 2. What is the impact of not going after that on you, those who love you, your community, and the world?

_____

_____

_____

_____

_____

4. What would you like to do about this?

_____

_____

_____

_____

5. How could you challenge yourself?

_____

_____

_____

_____

6. Who could hold you accountable?

_____

_____

_____

_____

Repeat questions 3 through 6 as many times as you'd like, using your answers in questions 1 and 2 to support your work.

THIS IS NOT A DIET: IT'S A LIFESTYLE

I am not one to preach perfection. I have a long way to go myself—and quite honestly, I know that I will never get there. And that's okay with me. Yet I want to add as much goodness into my day as possible and crowd out the not so good.

What's more important than eating perfectly healthfully is being a conscious eater. We need to recognize what's in every piece of food we put in our mouths, where it came from, and how it's going to make us feel. If we are okay with all of that, then I say go for that food. The problems happen when we don't even think about the foods we eat or understand why we look or feel the way we do. How can you make a conscious change when you aren't aware of what's wrong?

I have heard people refer to junk food as "garbage" or "poison," but I beg to differ. For me, something incredible happens when I pop a red Sour Patch Kid in my mouth. I'm transported back to fourth grade and a trip to the movie theater, sitting between my brother and sister, quietly unzipping my fanny pack to pull out my secret stash of candy. Slowly, I savor each sour gummy as *Free Willy* swims across the screen. It's

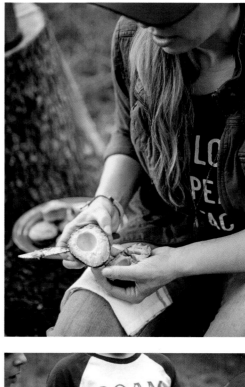

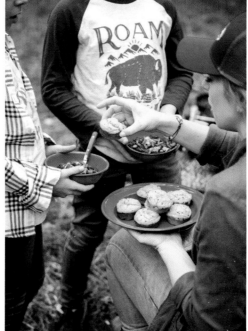

amazing to time travel just like that and get so much joy from a piece of candy.

Everyone has certain sugary, salty, or processed treats like my Sour Patch Kids that they just can't resist no matter how much they wish they could, but the key is moderation and being kind to yourself! Sure, it's harder to control the foods that contain addictive ingredients like processed sugars, "natural flavors," and caffeine. These ingredients are *anything* but natural, which is why it's so hard to put down the box, bag, or can until they are all gone.

I am not sharing this to get you to buy Sour Patch Kids or other junk foods "because Jen eats them." I'm doing it because I'd be lying to you if I didn't acknowledge that I enjoy candy at the movies or the Taco Bell drive-thru when we are on our way to my daughter's 3-hour gymnastics practice or the carryout pizza that gets dinner on the table after a particularly busy day. Some health advocates would rather starve than touch any of that "garbage," but not me. I enjoy every bite at that moment and thank the cashiers for helping me.

I also think about what I can do to make a better choice next time, because I know I can do better. Maybe I could have packed a snack and had it in the car before I took my daughter to gymnastics, or perhaps I could have stocked up on organic frozen pizza from the grocery store when it was on sale. Those would have been healthier options—and so I make an effort to pack the snacks and get those pizzas for the next time.

It's all about progress over perfection.

The more real, whole foods we eat, the more fabulous we will feel. So I'm committed to helping you eat more plants with a blender, a big salad bowl, a slow cooker, or straight outta the oven. If you need to squeeze in some pizza and ice cream in between, that's cool, too. Just remember: The more plant-powered foods you use to fuel your body, the more your body can fuel your passion.

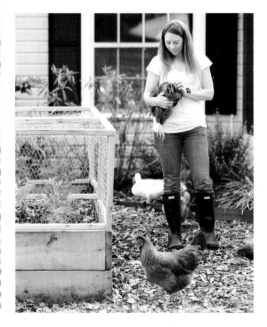

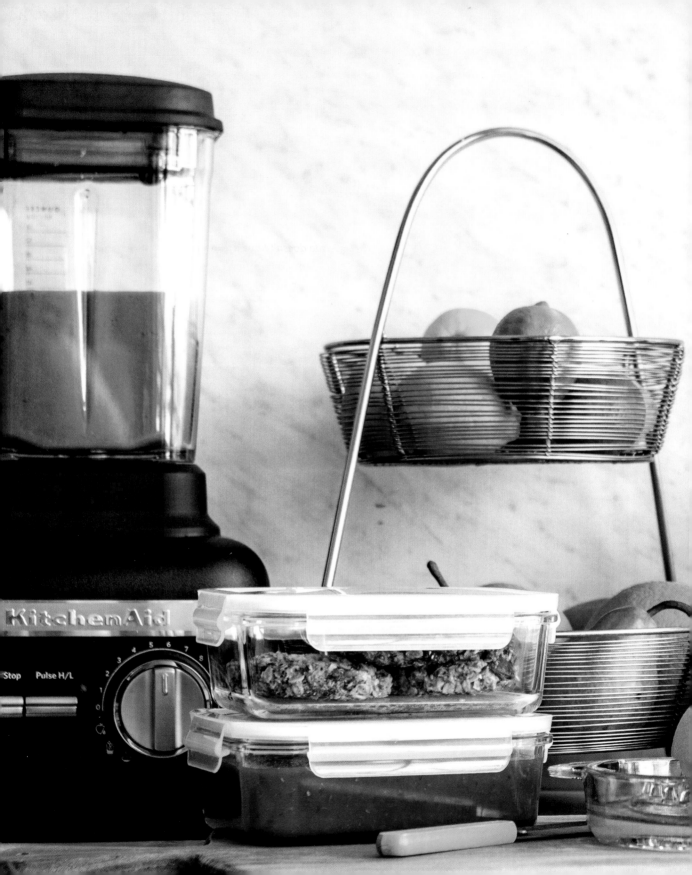

THE
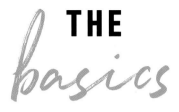
basics

An avocado doesn't have an ingredient list, an egg doesn't have a nutrition facts label, and an almond doesn't have a barcode. Eat food, not foodlike substances.

—MARK HYMAN, MD

Every year, a new diet or research study comes out claiming that some food is the enemy or the solution. It can be hard to know what's good for you and what's toxic. I cannot count the number of times coffee has been on the good list versus the bad list. I decided early on to choose my diet based not on what was trending or researched but rather on what made me feel best. There's no stronger lab to test foods than your own body. You don't have to be hard-core vegan to get big benefits from eating more plants. And you don't have to go cold Tofurky, either. Eating more plants can simply be an easy change here, a meatless Monday there. It all adds up to make a difference.

My philosophy is:

Eat more plants, however and whenever you can.

the simple eight
INGREDIENTS TO EMBRACE

I believe that embracing foods that come directly from nature and are minimally processed will help us thrive. The eight food groups below are the ones I embrace fully and try to source as much of my foods from as possible.

1 *fruits*

Fresh, whole fruits provide an instant, natural energy boost; prevent a number of diseases; satisfy a sweet tooth; and help you maintain glowing skin and healthy hair.

2 *veggies*

Veggies take care of our digestive, excretory, and skeletal systems as well as maintain blood pressure levels.

3 *leafy greens*

These are high in beneficial fiber and essential for burning fat, protecting brain cells, and maintaining a healthy heart.

4 *whole grains*

High in nutrients and fiber, whole grains lower the risk of serious diseases such as heart disease, stroke, diabetes, chronic inflammation, and cancer.

5 *legumes*

These are high in fiber and protein, which in turn help stabilize blood sugar levels and encourage weight loss.

6 *nuts and seeds*

Both are excellent sources of protein, healthy fats, and vitamin E, a powerful antioxidant that boosts skin health and the immune system. Some have high levels of omega-3 fatty acids, an essential fatty acid.

7 *dark chocolate*

As if you need another reason to eat dark chocolate, it promotes healthier skin and teeth, sharpens focus, and supports a healthy heart.

8 *healthy fats*

Healthy fats help curb hunger pangs and fuel long-term energy, plus they can strengthen the health of your eyes and skin.

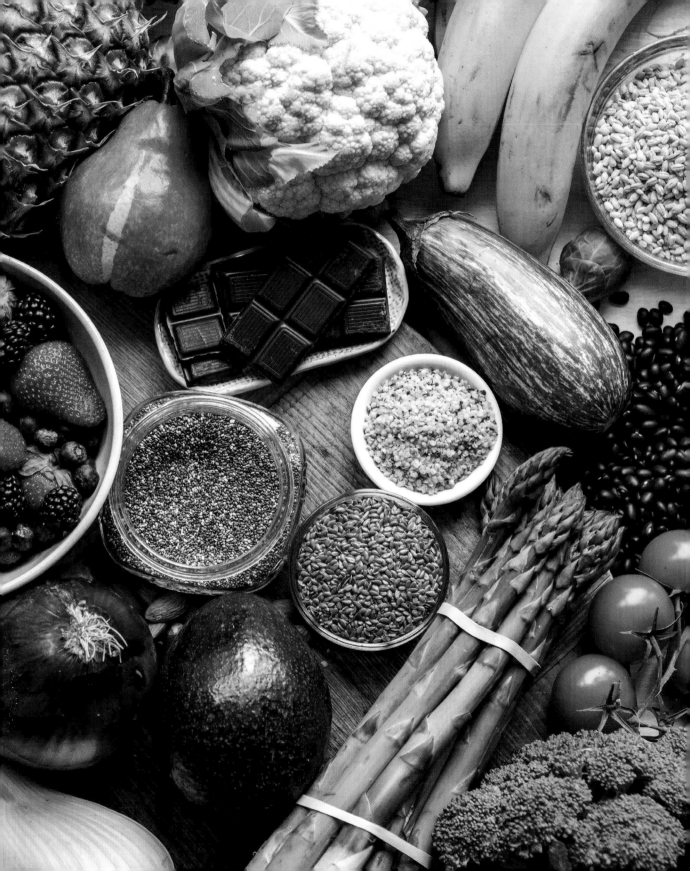

INGREDIENTS TO LIMIT

The foods we use as emotional crutches and artificial energy should be *limited*. Please note that I didn't say *avoided*, because that's not realistic for many of us. Yet moderation is what it's all about. Food additives, inflammation triggers, stimulants, and refined ingredients can drag your body down if you're not nourishing it with enough whole foods.

DAIRY

Dairy can be quite difficult to digest and is one of the most common triggers of food allergies. I recommend limiting dairy products and choosing organic, whole-fat products that are the least processed and contain the fewest additives. When it comes to butter, it's important to limit it as well, since it is still dairy. I recommend using grass-fed butter, which is made from cows that eat plants, which in turn yields high levels of omega-3s and vitamin A naturally.

REFINED SUGAR

Refined sugar is extracted from sugarcane or sugar beets in a process that creates a nutritionally void product. This type of sugar is acidic, highly addictive, and leaches nutrients from your body. Proven to contribute to mood problems, weight gain, and tooth decay, it also leads to spikes in blood sugar, leading to false "highs," followed by crashes in energy that leave you more tired than you were to begin with.

PROCESSED FOODS

As convenient as they are, processed foods provide very little in terms of nutrients. They place a burden on the liver and kidneys—the organs responsible for breaking down chemicals—making it harder for our bodies to function properly.

GLUTEN

Gluten (from the Latin term for glue) can create a sticky mess in the digestive tract. It can take significantly more energy for the body to digest gluten, and gluten also happens to be one of the most common food allergies because it can cause inflammation and irritable digestion. I recommend limiting the amount of gluten you consume, but it's not necessary to avoid it completely unless you are among those people who have a reaction to it.

CAFFEINE

As much as I love my daily cup of coffee, too much of a good thing can be harmful. Caffeine interferes with sleep, stresses the adrenal glands, and pillages our nutrient stores. It can create

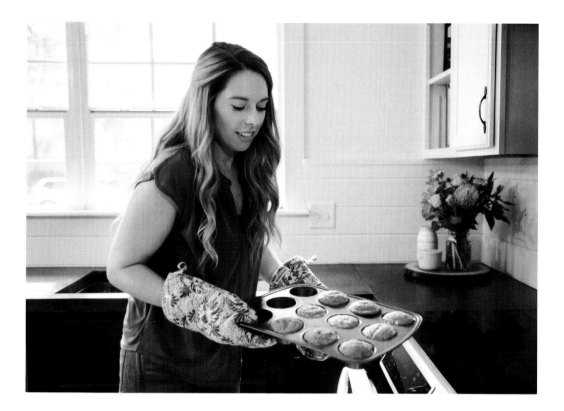

a false sense of energy, which can lead to adrenal fatigue over time. Yet caffeine is not the enemy—it just needs to be consumed in moderation (and early in the day) to reap the energy-boosting benefits.

ALCOHOL

In moderation, alcohol offers some health benefits, yet in large quantities, it's addictive, interferes with nutrient absorption, and is toxic to the liver. Alcohol can stimulate cravings for sugar and carbohydrates—which explains why you may find yourself craving that late-night pizza or find yourself elbow deep in a gallon of ice cream at the end of a night out.

SOY

I recommend staying away from highly processed soy products such as soy burgers and vegan chicken nuggets, because soy in its processed form can interfere with nutrient absorption and leach nutrients from your body. Consuming small amounts of organic, non-GM soy—such as tofu, miso, edamame, and tamari—is fine.

MEAT

As much as I advocate for my plant-based proteins, my husband and children just as strongly advocate for meat. When we have meat, I like to serve it alongside a plant-powered meal or as an optional topping to a hearty veggie bowl. Meat is highly acidic and can take up to 4 full days to move through your digestive system. This can cause digestive and skin issues, which is never fun. If you choose to eat meat, I suggest doing so in moderation and recommend purchasing 100 percent grass-fed and grass-finished beef, free-range organic chicken, wild-caught seafood, and nitrate-free pork.

EGGS

I've fallen in love with eggs since we started raising our own chickens and a duck. Farm-fresh eggs are incredibly delicious, high in protein, and a versatile ingredient in plant-based dishes. Eggs are high in cholesterol, however, and should be eaten in moderation.

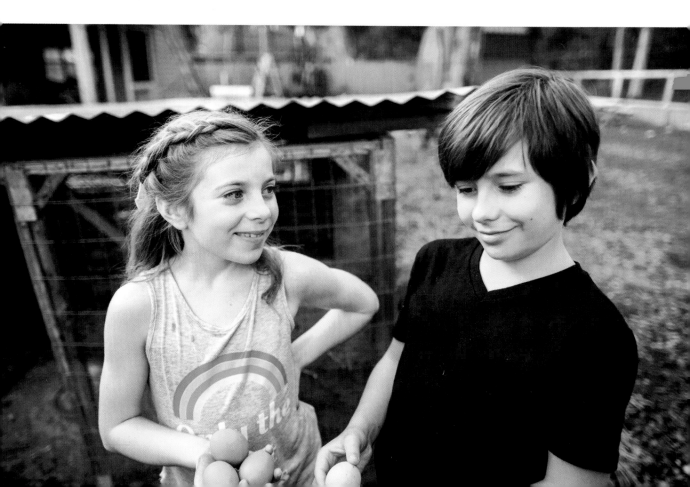

INGREDIENTS TO AVOID

The following items have no benefit to your health yet are found in many foods we buy at the grocery store. I suggest avoiding them as much as possible. But that doesn't mean you have to give up these ingredients 100 percent, because for most of us—myself included—that just isn't going to work. When I choose the occasional soda, candy, or chips, I know that these items are not going to benefit my body in any way. To counter that choice, I try to load up on nutrient-dense foods and hydrate my body to help flush out the toxins.

PROCESSED CORN

Corn syrup—also referred to as high fructose corn syrup, dextrose, or dextrin—is a cheap substitute for sugar that is used in soda and processed foods. High fructose corn syrup is incredibly difficult for your body to digest: It can take up to 4 days in comparison to the 24 hours your body needs to digest natural sugar.

FOOD COLORING

Multiple studies, including ones I have done on my own kids, show that eliminating food dyes reduces hyperactivity in young children. Additionally, the dyes Red 40, Yellow 5, and Yellow 6 have been found to contain cancer-causing contaminants.

MONOSODIUM GLUTAMATE (MSG)

Monosodium glutamate is a powerful flavor enhancer that activates the pleasure centers in the brain, making it highly addictive. If you have a hard time putting down the Chinese takeout or the fast-food burrito, there's a good chance it contains MSG.

ARTIFICIAL SWEETENERS

Aspartame is a low-calorie sweetener that has been linked to cancers and abnormal brain development. Sucralose is a chemical created in a labratory that is used to reduce the calorie count of foods while increasing their sweetness.

ARTIFICIAL FLAVORS

It says it right on the label: *"artificial flavoring"*—meaning it is fake, unnatural, and concocted in a chemistry lab to mimic natural flavors and trick your senses.

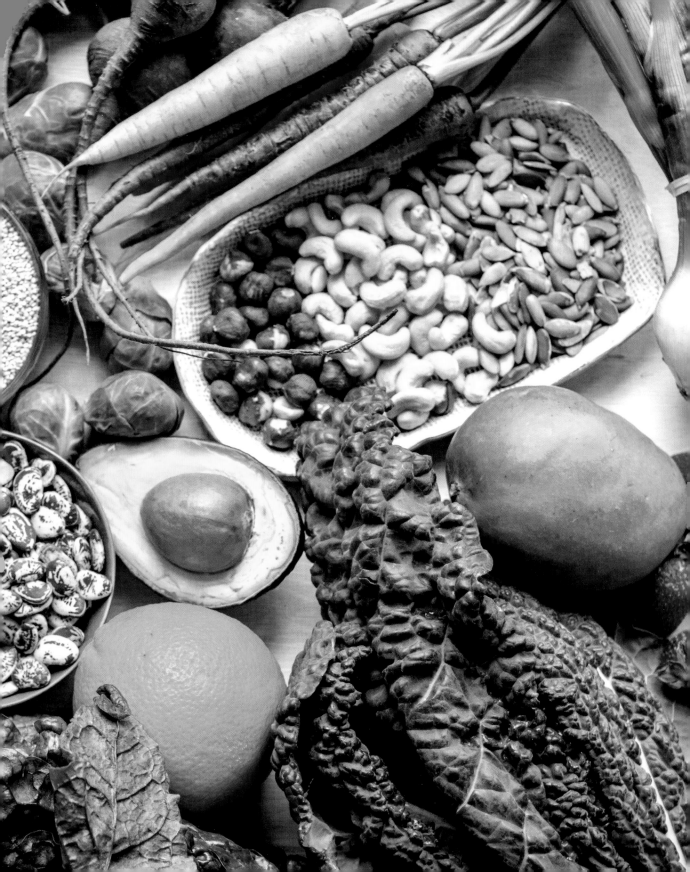

bottom line:
INVITE PLANTS TO EVERY MEAL

I've never been an advocate for changing everything overnight—it's better to focus on one small thing you can do today and do it well.

Over time, small daily changes and little victories lead to massive shifts. You can't blink and just say, "Adios ice cream and Snickers bars and hello kale chips and green smoothies." That would be setting yourself up for a quick relapse. Start by inviting plants to every meal. If you're buying ice cream, get one with real strawberries in it. If you're making grilled cheese, add a vegetable-based soup to the menu. You'll be surprised by how delicious that additional "guest" makes the meal, and soon you'll begin to crave it and the veggie portion size will increase.

Every recipe in this book invites a plant or two to the table . . . and oftentimes they are the guests of honor!

HOW I KEEP MY SANITY

I know it's not possible to make every meal from scratch and keep your sanity: Sometimes food just needs to end up on the table. So when you're hitting the store for shortcut items—like bread, tortillas, tomato sauce, ketchup, and other staples—remember that reading the label is key to avoiding the ingredients that are more harmful than good. Doing research can feel daunting at first, but it really does get easier as you do it more. A shortcut that I use is looking for items that are certified organic, which will rule out all the harmful ingredients listed in this section. I also recommend choosing foods that contain five ingredients or fewer. For example, buy the popcorn that is just corn, oil, and salt. Once you find the brand that works for you, it's easy to pick it up the next time.

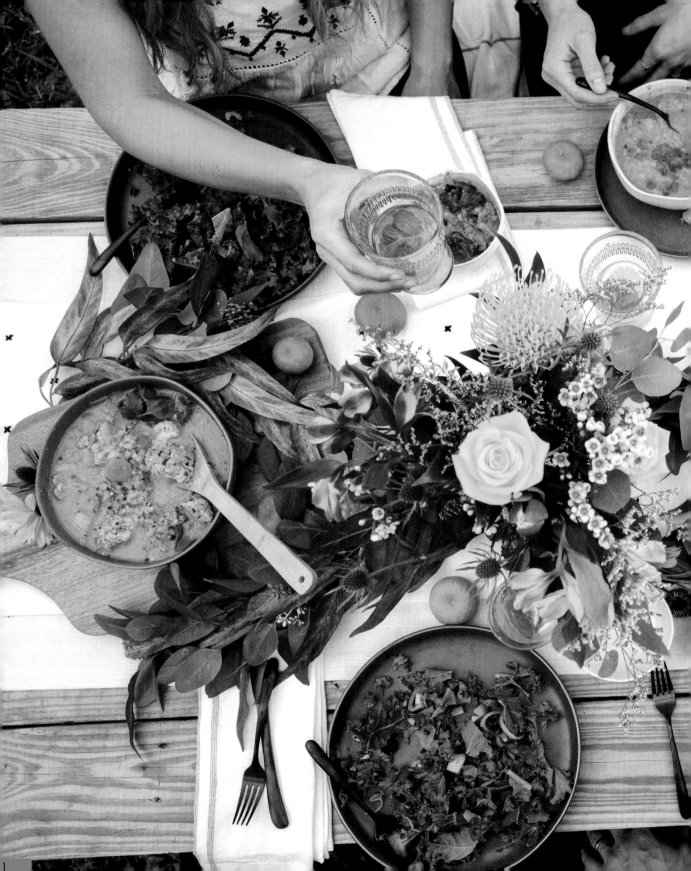

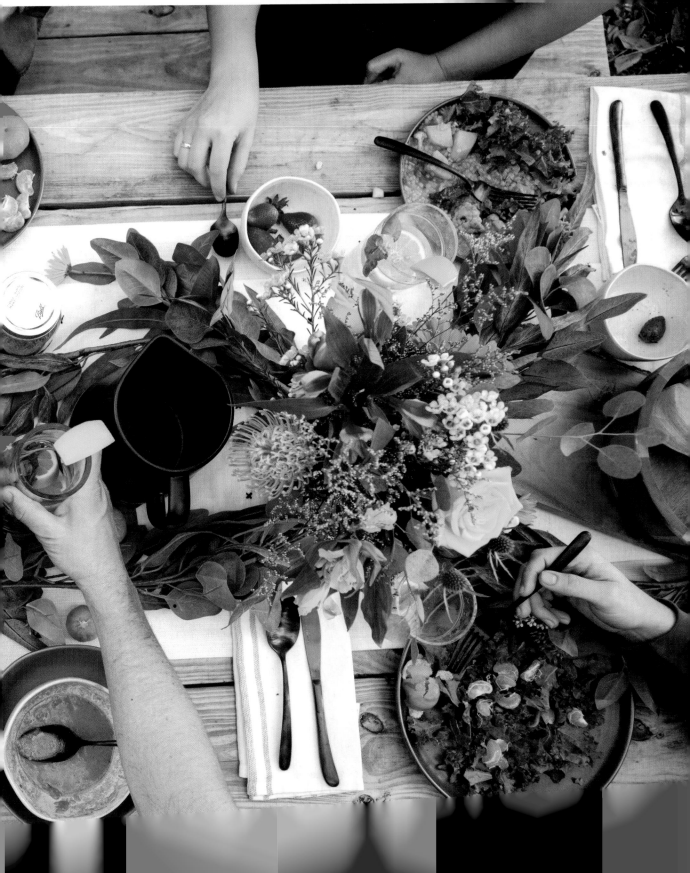

meet the rawkstars

ROXANA HAZRAT

Adding plant-based recipes and whole foods to my diet has been an amazingly positive experience. As someone who already loves to cook and eat vegetables and whole foods, I wasn't expecting much of a change, but I have found that adding more plant-based recipes to my regular meal rotation has improved my overall health, including my mood, energy levels, and even weight management.

ELSIE KIBUE–NGARE

My eating habits have definitely changed for the best, and the fact that my ever-so-reluctant husband joined me in one of the cleanses with surprising results is a huge win in my book, proving that I am glad to have come across Simple Green Smoothies. My little daily triumphs from all of this are seeing my family enjoy some of the meals I make from SGS, with little tweaks here and there.

KAREN WIEDMEIER

I've been a vegetarian for most of my life, for ethical reasons. In my twenties, I could get away with eating pretty much anything—and trust me, there is plenty of unhealthy vegetarian/vegan food around. As I got older, my body didn't bounce back from bad eating the way it used to, and even though my diet was vegan, I wasn't feeling the best. Who would feel great, eating a steady stream of highly processed food? Enter Simple Green Smoothies! This was the answer—plant-based, whole-food recipes that broke my cravings for all the processed, "carby" foods. The online cleanses laid everything out so precisely that there was no way I could fail . . . and the group support kept me on track. I love that this way of eating is not a fad—it's just healthy, whole-plant foods . . . and everything is so delicious! At 58, my energy is high, my sleep is improved, and weight loss happens naturally. I'm so glad I found SGS . . . it's made my life better in so many ways!

HOLLY COUCH

In 2017, I did the Fresh Start: A 21-Day Cleanse from Simple Green Smoothies. I was determined to stick it out—and honestly, this was a turning point for me. After 21 days of whole-food, plant-based eating, I felt like a new person. I felt incredible! Health issues that I had been dealing with for years (that I didn't even know were issues—I just thought they were normal for everyone) subsided. I didn't have the cravings I normally had. I got so many compliments from people about how I looked (not just about weight loss but about glowing skin and the overall appearance of great health). I was also more aware of how each food affected my body after reintroducing it into my meals and was able to pinpoint those that caused me trouble. Since finishing the cleanse, I have maintained a plant-based diet 90 percent of the time. I occasionally eat meat. I occasionally enjoy a little too much bread. I still love chocolate. But I don't feel tied down by those things anymore because I know how incredible I feel when I'm eating well. I'm never too tempted to keep indulging (and when I am, I jump back into Simple Green Smoothies Thrive: 7-Day Reset) because I know I feel like the best version of myself when I'm eating a healthy, plant-based diet. I have Simple Green Smoothies to thank for that!

— — — — — — — — — — — — — — — — —

GENEVIEVE MOREHEAD

Starting this plant-based journey, I was hoping for a little more balance in my life but wasn't expecting much. My health was good (though my weight was not). I had a decent amount of energy and a fairly balanced diet. My kids ate well, though more easy/quick food than I would prefer, but it wasn't "too much." Simple Green Smoothies came into our lives and turned my world upside down in the best way. My weight started to drop off without any outward effort, my panels at the doctor went from "in range mostly" to "What are you doing?! They're perfect!," my energy soared, my kids and husband are willingly (and happily) eating plates full of plant-based deliciousness. My meat-and-potatoes husband even asks for leftovers for lunch instead of the meat-centric meals he can get at work. Simple Green Smoothies not only helped bring more balance and nutrition in the form of truly delicious food to my table but has given me the confidence to continue to feed myself and my family the best foods with the most amazing flavors. SGS has made my world a much greener and delicious place, and I can't wait to add this book to my life.

— — — — — — — — — — — — — — — — —

SANDI O'DONNELL

In just 3 months of embracing Simple Green Smoothies plant-based recipes, I have noticed drastic changes to my body. Since then, I have lost 12 pounds (so far) without ever feeling hungry or deprived! Every week my body naturally sheds 1 to 2 pounds without my really having to work on it. I no longer have pain in my joints, my skin looks amazing, and I have so much more energy! I see food differently and now understand that it is fuel for my body, and I treat myself with fresh fruits and berries as dessert instead of my previous sugar choices. For the first time, I am looking forward to going in for my yearly with my naturopath, as I am excited to show her how far I have come in just a couple of short months! I feel empowered and excited for the future! Simple Green Smoothies is such a great group, and I feel like I have finally found my tribe!

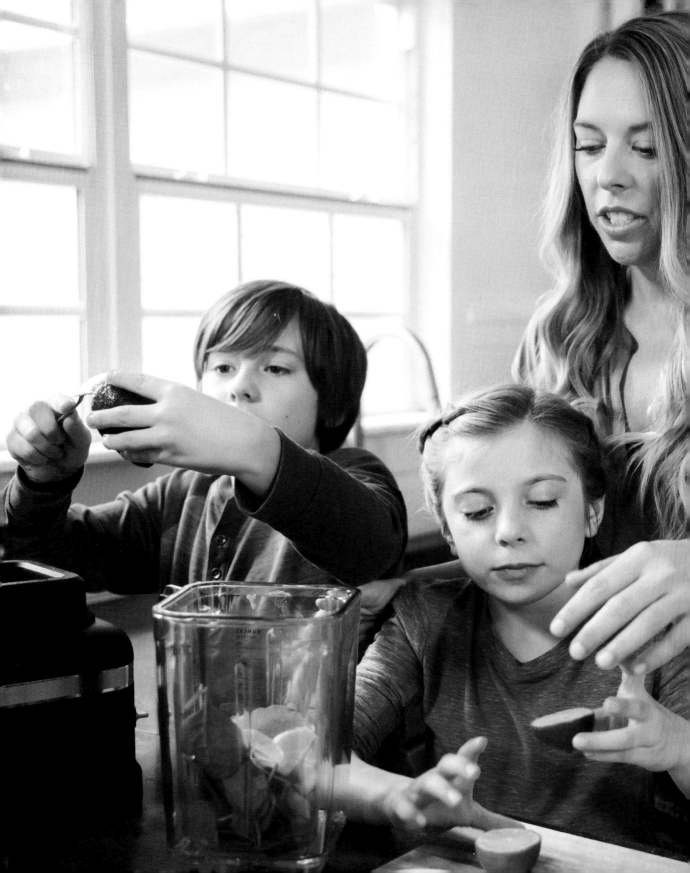

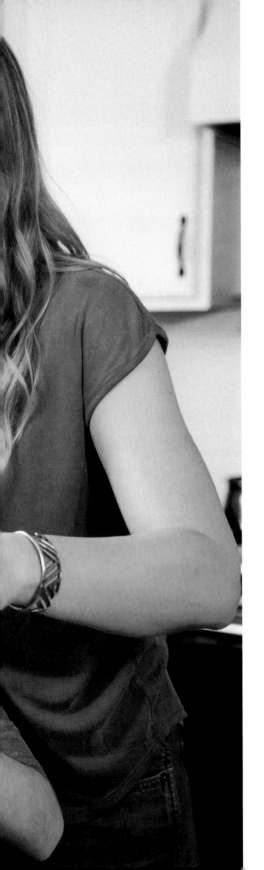

MAKING IT
work

There are resources galore when it comes to eating healthy. Blogs, social media, magazines, books, restaurants, and scientific journals are filled with inspiration and information if you only look. Yet the truth is, it's just too much to handle! You can take in only so much air before you have to exhale it out, and it's the same with information in the wellness sector.

So rather than shove it all down your throat, I thought we could go step by step through the main pieces of advice that have kept me sane and eating healthier than ever.

SHOP CONFIDENTLY

I enjoy shopping, but I don't love it. For example, Target is great because I can buy groceries, Halloween costumes, makeup, toilet paper, and a new outfit all in one checkout. I'm that person who comes to the register with the cart overflowing on all sides with adorable throw pillows piled high on top of my bananas, underwear, and the dress that was 20 percent off with a coupon. That's my kind of shopping—hit it once and hit it good.

There was a time when it took me 2 hours to get through the grocery aisles because I would read every label before putting an item in my cart. I remember gasping when I learned the ketchup brand we used daily contained high fructose corn syrup, which I had been giving to my corn-sensitive toddler. Food is medicine, and I was giving my son a food that was making him sick. I've come a long way since then!

The good news is that grocery stores have changed *a lot* since 2009. Organic food is quite mainstream now, making label reading and decision making much easier. Coconut oil can be found in practically every store out there, including pet stores, strangely enough!

THE BIG THREE

Here's a cheat sheet to help you get started shopping confidently. Start small and make progress every day. From here, you'll be able to build out your plant-powered whole-foods kitchen.

the big three deal makers

These are the top three claims on the front of food packaging that I embrace.

1. Organic
2. Non-GMO
3. Unsweetened

the big three deal breakers

These are the top three ingredients listed on food labels that I avoid.

1. Corn syrup
2. Food dye
3. Artificial sugars

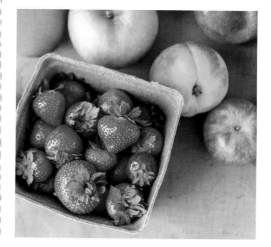

a guide to buying produce . . . and saving money

More than once, I have spent 5 minutes staring down apples in the grocery store, debating with myself which ones to buy. Organic for $2 more, or nonorganic for $2 less? It can be stressful when you're trying to eat healthfully on a budget! The thing that saved me is when I learned about the Dirty Dozen report released annually by the Environmental Working Group (EWG).

I use the EWG report to help me decide what to buy organic and what isn't as important—which can save money and sanity when staring down the apples.

EWG'S DIRTY DOZEN

This is a list of the produce that has the highest levels of contamination from pesticides, meaning that these are the items you may want to prioritize when you decide which foods to buy organic.

1. Strawberries
2. Spinach
3. Nectarines
4. Apples
5. Grapes
6. Peaches
7. Cherries
8. Pears
9. Tomatoes
10. Celery
11. Potatoes
12. Bell peppers and hot peppers

EWG'S CLEAN 15

This list includes produce that is least likely to be contaminated by pesticides. These are ones that you can buy safely without the organic label.

1. Avocados
2. Sweet corn*
3. Pineapples
4. Cabbage
5. Onions
6. Frozen sweet peas
7. Papayas*
8. Asparagus
9. Mangoes
10. Eggplant
11. Honeydew
12. Kiwifruit
13. Cantaloupe
14. Cauliflower
15. Broccoli

*Some of the sweet corn and papaya sold in the United States is genetically modified. Purchase organic for these crops if you have a choice.

grocery store staples guide

To make shopping as easy as possible, I've compiled a list of the staple items I buy and use throughout this recipe book. If you're ready to wipe the slate clean and start fresh, this list will give you a solid foundation to healthy eating. This list is also your permission slip to ditch the random specialty stuff and embrace a simple, healthy life.

DAIRY & EGGS

Almond milk (unsweetened), eggs (organic, free-range), grass-fed butter

FRUITS *(buy based on season and availability)*

Apples, apricots, avocados, bananas, blueberries, cherries, lemons, mangoes, melons, oranges, peaches, pears, pineapple, pomegranates, raspberries, strawberries, watermelons

HEALTHY FATS

Avocado oil, organic virgin coconut oil, extra-virgin olive oil, sesame oil, MCT oil

DRIED FRUIT & NUTS

Almonds, apricots, cashews, cherries, cranberries, dates, raisins

BAKING ITEMS

Almond meal, coconut flour, vegan chocolate chips, gluten-free flour, gluten-free rolled oats, unbleached all-purpose flour, whole wheat flour

FREEZER

Frozen fruit (blueberries, mangoes, peaches, pineapple, strawberries), veggies (green beans, peas)

VEGGIES *(buy based on season and availability)*

Asparagus, broccoli, Brussels sprouts, carrots, cauliflower, cherry tomatoes, green beans, kale, spinach, sweet potatoes, yellow onions, zucchini

SWEETENERS

Pure maple syrup, honey

SUPERFOODS

Chia seeds, hemp hearts, nutritional yeast, plant-based protein powder (unsweetened)

PANTRY ITEMS

Apple cider vinegar (with the mother), black beans, brown rice, chickpeas, coconut milk, curry paste, kidney beans, lentils (dried), pumpkin puree, quinoa, vegetable stock, tahini, organic canned tomatoes, pure vanilla extract

HERBS & SPICES

Basil, black pepper, cilantro, cinnamon, curry powder, fennel, garlic, ginger, ground red pepper, Himalayan sea salt, Italian seasoning, mint, paprika, turmeric; Frank's RedHot, ketchup, Sriracha sauce, tamari

KEEP COSTS DOWN

When I started getting into healthy, whole foods, my family was in a tough spot financially. We had moved across the country for my husband's new job as a pastor of a church plant. Within a year, the church plant closed down, and we were barely making ends meet with unemployment checks, help from my parents, and income from our freelance jobs. Our health insurance had just expired, and we were receiving WIC checks to help pay for groceries for our kids, who were 2 and 3 years old at the time. I was always scared that one of the kids would get sick and we'd end up in the emergency room with a hefty bill that we couldn't afford.

I took our family's health into my own hands and started blending a daily green smoothie to nourish our bodies and boost our immune systems. I was able to buy some of the smoothie supplies with the WIC vouchers and afforded the rest by cutting spending in other areas. As financially strapped as we were, I knew that we couldn't sacrifice our health. It's just not worth it. Here's what else we did to make nutritious foods a priority in our home—and these strategies may work in yours.

TIP 1: MAKE SIMPLE SWAPS

When changing your diet, you don't have to buy everything I—or anyone else—recommend. Swap one item you are currently using for a better one, one at a time if that's what it takes to make this work for you. Over the years, I've been inspired by so many wellness advocates, from Danielle Walker to Mark Hyman to Angela Liddon to Melissa Hartwig. I've adjusted the way I eat to an approach that works best for me. Which is a bit of a mosaic.

Here are simple swaps that you can gradually build into your pantry and into your routine.

	REPLACE WITH
Vegetable oil	Organic virgin coconut oil
Table salt	Unrefined sea salt
Cow's milk	Unsweetened almond milk
Refined sugar	Maple syrup
Soy sauce	Tamari
White rice	Brown rice
Soda	Water (or kombucha, for a sweet tooth)
Candy bar	Trail mix (or unsweetened dried fruit)

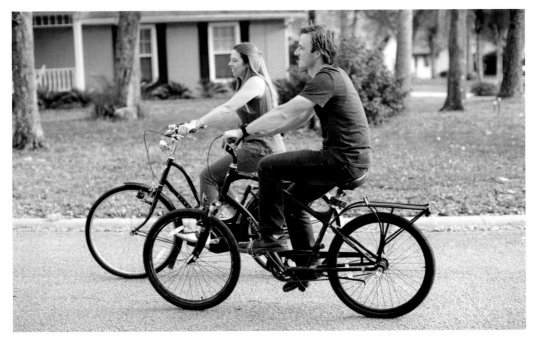

To cut expenses, we swapped our truck for bikes and use them as much as possible.

TIP 2: INVEST IN A WHOLESALE CLUB MEMBERSHIP

There are so many wholesale membership options out there now. My favorites are ThriveMarket.com, Costco, and Amazon Subscribe & Save, which have a great range of organic and high-quality ingredients at a fraction of the price of my local grocery store.

TIP 3: MEAL PREP

We originally started to prep our meals for our sanity, but we've cut back on food waste as well. The amount of money prep saves you in groceries is amazing! I don't know about you, but we used to throw out tons of rotten food that we'd buy yet not get around to eating before it went bad. Planning your grocery list around a specific set of meals and snacks is a great way to purchase only what you plan to use.

TIP 4: SHOP SEASONALLY

I have always been a bargain shopper and learned early that the best deals on produce are those that are freshest and in abundance. Down here in Florida, strawberries are in season every March and drop to $1 a pound, sometimes less if we hit a farmstand! Grocery stores put a higher price on out-of-season items because those foods are harder to find, there is higher demand, and also because out-of-season foods have to be shipped from farther away.

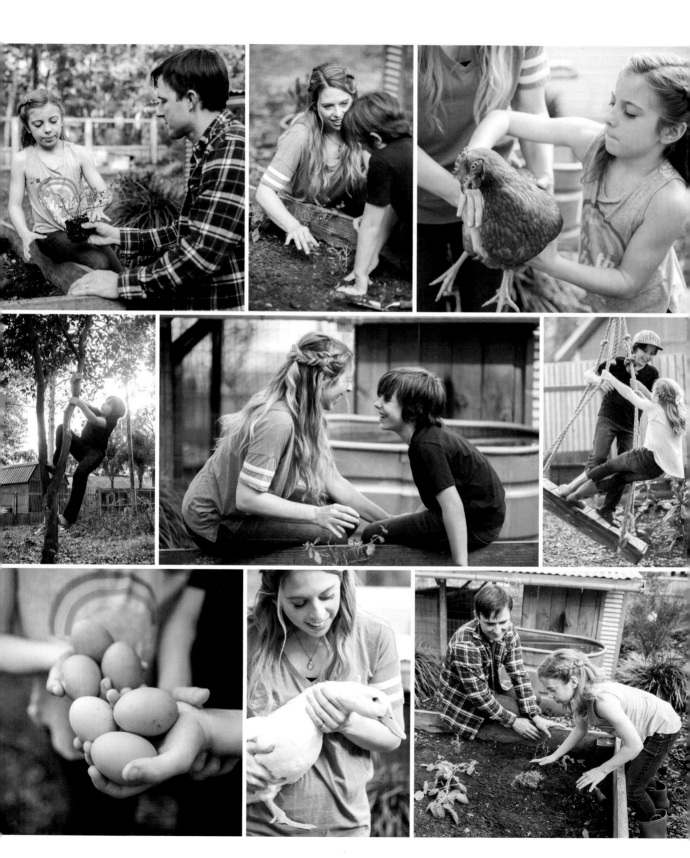

TIP 5: GROW YOUR OWN

If you are passionate, driven, and have a green thumb, you can grow your own food and save money. Yet I have to be honest, after three growing seasons, I don't believe we've recouped the cost of the lumber to build our raised garden beds here at Hansard Farm. So if you're thinking of growing your own garden to save money, you have to really be motivated and on top of it. To yield a harvest that can make it a savings takes a lot of work! We do it for the joy of the experience and for our kids to understand where food comes from and how we can cut down on waste by composting and then using the compost as nutrients for our plants.

TRAVEL SMART

Eating healthy is super hard when traveling. There, I said it. I've lost the clean-eating battle many times on the road, especially when we visit the West Coast (our homeland) and pass an In-N-Out Burger. And I'm totally fine with that! Making one healthy choice a day is what we strive for. That's it. So I'll blend a green smoothie for breakfast and head on over to In-N-Out for lunch (and enjoy every bite!).

But if you're looking for travel-smart ideas, here are healthy choices for your times on the road.

TIP 1: GET IN THAT GREEN SMOOTHIE

I try to get in a daily green smoothie while away from home. Sometimes this is the only healthy thing I'll have all day. But it's better than nothing. If I have space in my luggage, I've been known to pack a small blender and whip up a smoothie in my hotel room. Other times, I'll find a local smoothie or juice bar.

TIP 2: DO RESTAURANT RESEARCH

I jump on Yelp and look for a good "burger joint," "taco truck," or "farm-to-table restaurant." Typically I can scour a menu and find an awesome veggie burger, sweet potato fries, and guacamole and be in my happy place. Or I can revamp a chicken fajita taco into one with black beans, onions, and green peppers. You simply have to be willing to ask someone to help you out—people almost always have really cool ideas and enjoy getting creative with me. Just remember to be polite and tip well when your server puts in the extra effort!

adventure is out there!

Traveling has been one of the greatest blessings in my life. My first memory of traveling was when I was 2 years old (no joke!) and my dad took me on an airplane from Los Angeles to New York. I remember looking out the window, being in awe of all the little cute houses below. Visiting different places has allowed me to meet many incredible people and taste so many amazing foods. I strongly encourage you to take a little adventure of your own.

Here are more ideas:

STAY LOCAL. Spend the day exploring your own town in a whole new way by geocaching. With GPS coordinate clues, you can find hidden "caches"—usually a box with a logbook inside—in places you didn't even know existed in your town. You can learn more at geocaching.com.

GET IN NATURE. Scout out a state or national park or forest that piques your interest. Pick a hiking trail and go for it. Make sure to pack some granola bars, trail mix, apples, and lots of water!

BE A FOODIE. Head to a big city and sign up for a local food tour. You'll learn more about the culture, the chefs, the foods, and the flavors than you ever thought possible.

CHILLAX. Head to a lake or the beach or a river—just get by water and allow the natural sounds soothe and calm you. Water is such great therapy! Bring a blanket, some healthy snacks, and a book you've been wanting to read.

SAY YES TO ADVENTURE. Find a local rock-climbing gym and take a rappelling lesson. Go whitewater rafting. Take a hot-air balloon ride. Hike to a waterfall and stand beneath the spray.

TRANSPORT YOURSELF. Go somewhere you don't speak the language and have never been before. Be open to your new surroundings, smile at strangers, jump on a city bus or take a tuk-tuk, and taste foods you've never sampled.

TIP 3: GROCERY SHOP

I try to scout out a Trader Joe's or Whole Foods Market when I'm traveling. I grab a few simple snacks to hold me over. My regulars are kombucha, nuts, guacamole, hummus, sweet potato chips, carrots, and trail mix.

TIP 4: DO YOUR BEST, AND FORGET THE REST

This phrase is what my son's preschool teacher would tell the kids. Over the years, it's stuck with me, and I hear myself saying it whenever I feel like I've messed up. The fact that we are even able to make any healthy choices in our world of fast and quick is pretty remarkable. As much focus as I put on eating food that nourishes my body, I also believe in creating memorable experiences. If that means grabbing a slice of pizza three days in a row on a NYC corner with my kids, I will do it. And have! If that means going out for ice cream at Salt & Straw in Portland after a day on the river, we are there! The point is: Don't beat yourself up! Find the good that is in everything. It's there, I promise.

USE PROPER TOOLS

I like to keep my kitchen as simple as possible, which means if a tool isn't being used, it doesn't stick around for long. The ones below have become staples in my kitchen; I'd have a hard time getting through a week without them.

BLENDER. This is the most-used appliance by far in my kitchen. I use it for blending smoothies, frothing hot beverages, chopping veggies, pureeing soups, and grinding almonds into butter. I recommend purchasing a high-powered one with a great warranty. Check out my blender guide for more advice: http://sgs.to/blenders.

SPIRALIZER. Turning zucchini into zoodles and sweet potatoes into swoodles—I am so thankful someone created this creative contraption!

MANUAL JUICER. A manual juicer is simple to use and saves your hands from the acidic juice as well as limits the amount of wayward squirts.

FOOD PROCESSOR. I used to think my blender could do everything, but I was wrong when it comes to chopping small amounts of things like garlic, onions, and nuts and especially when it comes to making pesto. I tried making pesto in my blender—the blender was so powerful that the "pesto" turned to slime. Now I stick with the food processor.

GLASS STORAGE. These containers are great for storing food and using as meal prep. The glass allows them to be frozen, baked, and refrigerated, which saves a dish or two.

TOTE BAGS. Every trip to the market deserves a cute tote bag. I like to keep my bags in my trunk (my friend Erin taught me that one) and have them ready to go when I'm shopping.

GOOD KNIFE. Once I almost cut my fingers off with a dull blade while chopping a watermelon. The duller the knife is, the more pressure you have to use to make a cut and the more out of control it gets. Trust me—your precious hands are worth a new, sharp knife.

FRUIT BASKET. Having a countertop container to display your fruit in is a must if you're trying to eat more plants. We like to keep oranges, mangos, avocado, plums, and pears in our fruit basket for a quick grab-and-go snack.

RICE COOKER. The first time I saw a rice cooker was when a friend was making macaroni and cheese in it. That was the day I vowed to own one someday. The funny thing is, I have never made mac-and-cheese in mine, yet we do cook a lot of rice and quinoa in it! I love that the cooker can be set ahead of time and the food will stay warm for hours. I'll set the cooker on, then I can focus completely on roasting the veggies and frying the eggs as my trusty little cooker goes to work.

MASON JARS. I truly can't imagine life without these things! We use them as drinking cups in our house, as well as water bottles, granola and nut storage, and leftover smoothie holders.

SLOW COOKER. Using this convenient appliance is a great way to get dinner taken care of at 8:00 a.m., when you are still fresh.

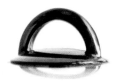

STOP COUNTING CALORIES— I MEAN IT!

When we think of food as numbers, it zaps the joy that is in a meal. The flavors, the crunch, the aromas, the nutrients, the hydration, the fuel—this is what food is all about! So rather than counting calories, I focus on eating foods that will give me the things I want and celebrate that! I want to be strong and energized so I can go after the activities that matter most to me. Which is playing baseball with my son, riding bikes with my daughter, trail running with a friend, and doing obstacle course races with my husband. That's why I decide to eat food that can be high-quality fuel.

The simple truth is that all calories are not equal. You can gulp down a cup of soda or a cup of green smoothie, and—while the calories are similar—the amount of sugar and the percentage of recommended dietary allowance are going to be dramatically different.

If weight loss is a goal, you can happily achieve this without counting calories. When you focus on nutrients instead of calories, that's when the momentum begins.

I've shared a ton of tips to help you add more plants and whole foods into your diet. Remember, you don't have to do them all at once. Focus on a few at a time until they become habits, then up your plant-powered game. In the next section, I'll show you how to overhaul your diet with amazing plant-based recipes—one meal at a time.

You got this!

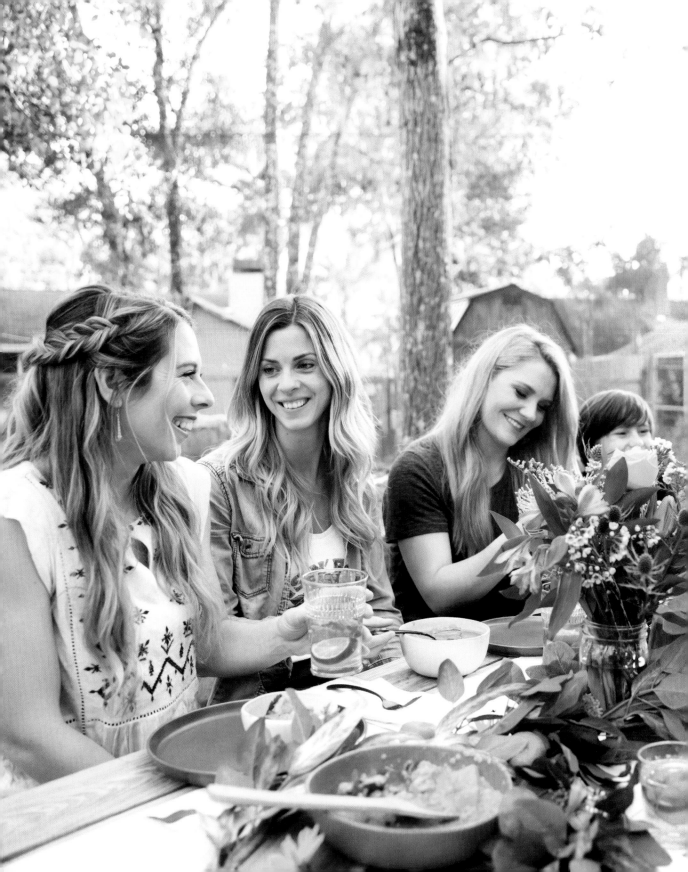

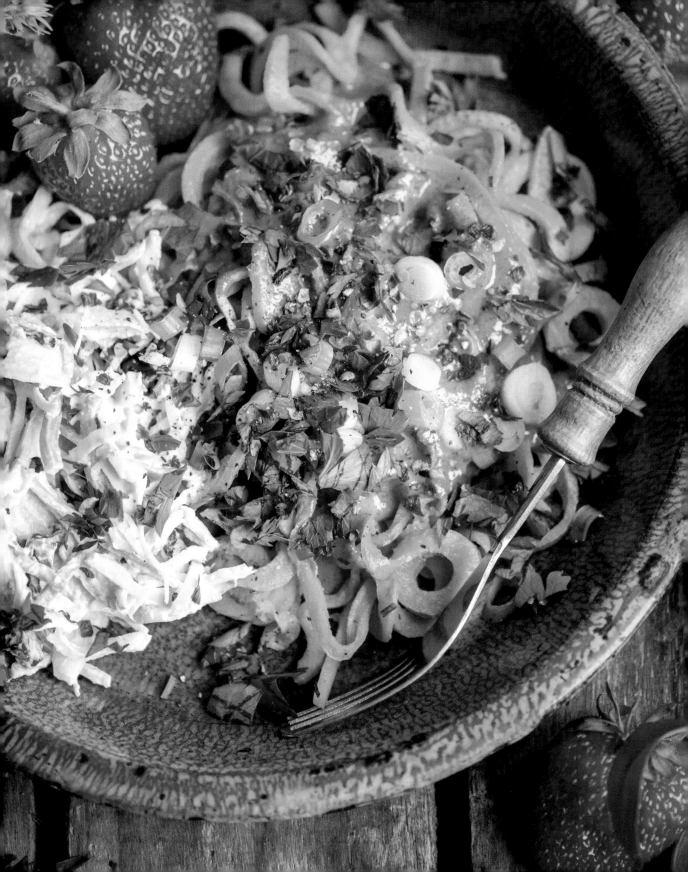

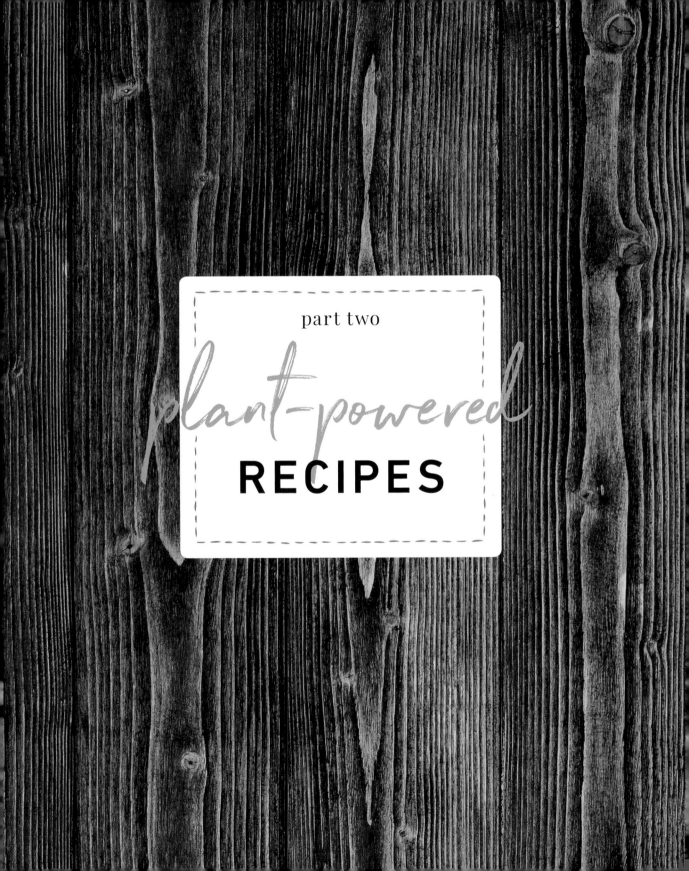

part two

plant-powered

RECIPES

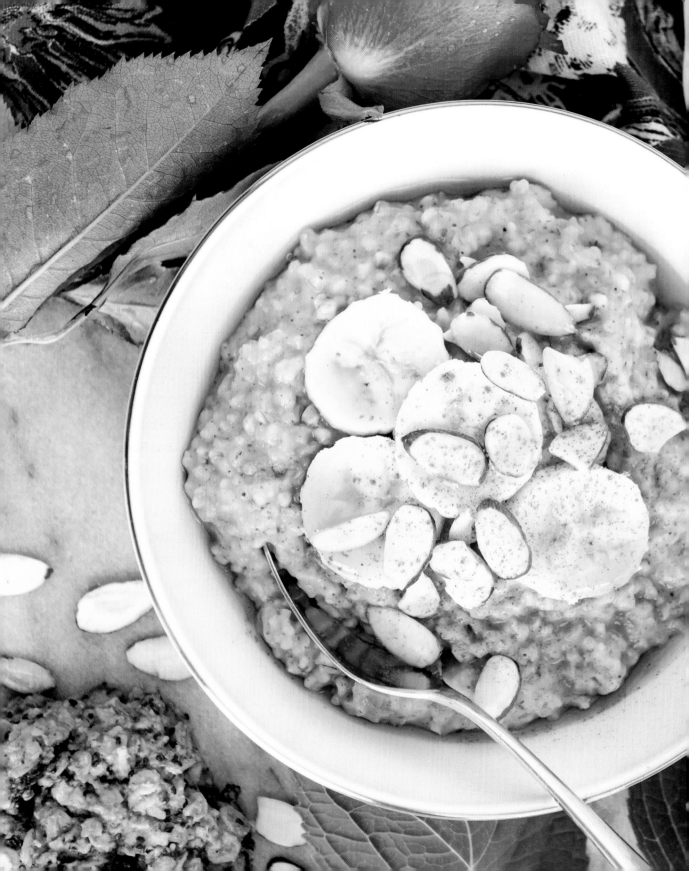

breakfasts

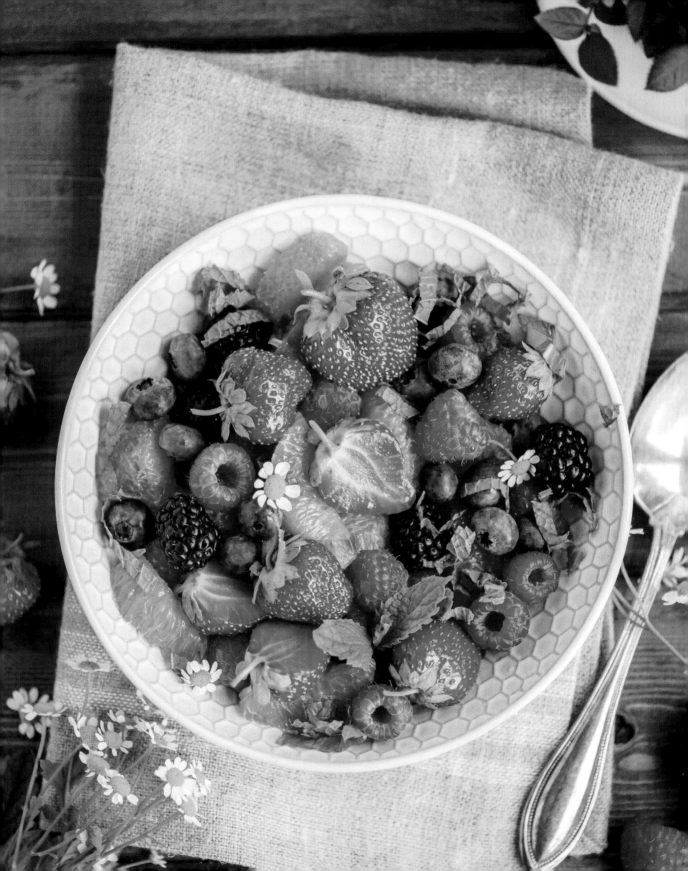

spring breakfast salad

When I was pregnant with my son, Jackson, I craved fast-food hamburgers and fresh citrus. I was a die-hard vegetarian back then, so I never gave in to the burgers, but I sure did eat a whole lot of oranges, grapefruit, and lemons. Yes, I even ate lemons . . . like oranges. This bright citrus-berry breakfast bowl stems from that time and has become one of my son's favorite fruit salads. Go figure. **SERVES 2**

½ cup strawberries
½ cup blueberries
½ cup blackberries
½ cup raspberries
1 grapefruit, peeled and segmented

3 tablespoons fresh orange juice (from 1 orange)
1 tablespoon pure maple syrup
¼ cup chopped fresh mint
¼ cup sliced almonds

1. In a serving bowl, combine the berries and grapefruit.

2. In a small bowl, stir together the orange juice and maple syrup. Pour the syrup mixture over the fruit. Sprinkle with the mint and almonds. Serve immediately.

- -

GLUTEN FREE, NUT FREE *(remove nuts)*, VEGAN, DAIRY FREE

spiced baked oatmeal

When the temperature dropped and the fall winds came blowing through his Idaho town, my husband's Grandpa Laws would start each morning with oatmeal. He did this every single day until the weather turned to spring. Then he would put the oatmeal away until the next fall. Talk about a man with healthy habits! Whenever I eat oatmeal, I fondly think of him. He passed away years ago, but his traditions and loving spirit are still felt in our family. This comforting, warm oatmeal recipe is in honor of him. SERVES 6

2 tablespoons organic virgin coconut oil, melted, plus a little more for greasing the pan
3 ripe pears, cored and diced
2 cups unsweetened plain almond milk
¼ cup pure maple syrup
1 tablespoon pure vanilla extract

2 cups gluten-free rolled oats
¾ cup chopped pecans
½ cup raisins
1 teaspoon ground cinnamon
½ teaspoon ground ginger
¼ teaspoon ground nutmeg
¼ teaspoon sea salt

1. Preheat the oven to 350°F. Grease a 13 × 9-inch baking dish with a little oil. Evenly distribute the pears in the bottom of the pan.

2. In a medium bowl, whisk together the almond milk, maple syrup, vanilla, and melted oil.

3. In a large bowl, stir together the oats, pecans, raisins, cinnamon, ginger, nutmeg, and salt. Add the almond milk mixture and stir well. Spread evenly over the pears.

4. Bake for 30 to 40 minutes, or until the center is set.

- -

GLUTEN FREE, NUT FREE (remove nuts and replace almond milk with coconut milk), VEGAN, DAIRY FREE

rawkstar tip

SWAP IT UP: Apples can be used in place of pears, and any nut can be substituted for the pecans. Try other dried fruits such as cherries, blueberries, currants, apricots, or cranberries instead of raisins.

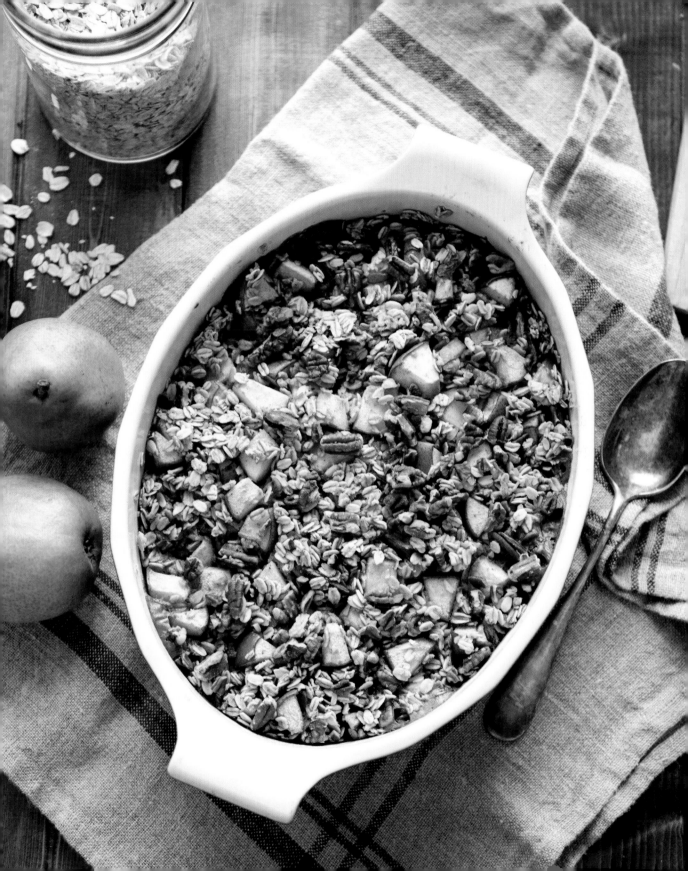

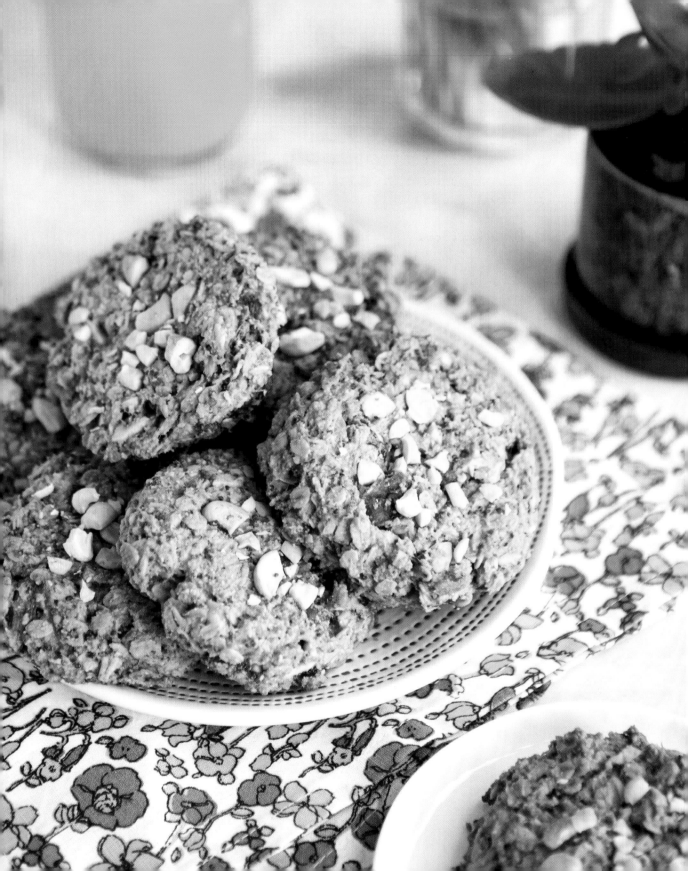

morning glory cookies

Who doesn't want a cookie for breakfast?! I fell in love with them when I realized how much protein and flavor could be packed into a single cookie! These are great for an on-the-go breakfast or as a preworkout snack. I grab one (or two!) before I hit the trail for a long run.

MAKES 12 LARGE COOKIES

2 cups gluten-free rolled oats
1 cup almond flour
¼ cup chia seeds
1 teaspoon baking soda
½ teaspoon ground cinnamon
½ teaspoon sea salt
1 cup mashed ripe banana

½ cup cashew butter
¼ cup organic virgin coconut oil, melted
1 teaspoon pure vanilla extract
¾ cup pitted dates, chopped
½ cup unsweetened shredded coconut
½ cup raw cashews, chopped

1. Preheat the oven to 350°F. Line 2 baking sheets with parchment paper.

2. In a large mixing bowl, stir together the oats, almond flour or meal, chia seeds, baking soda, cinnamon, and salt. In another bowl, combine the banana, cashew butter, oil, and vanilla.

3. Make a well in the center of the oats mixture. Pour the banana mixture into the well and stir until thoroughly combined. Fold in the dates, coconut, and cashews.

4. Using a ⅓-cup measuring cup, drop small mounds of the dough onto the baking sheets, leaving a little space between each mound. There should be 12 large cookies. Gently press on the tops to flatten slightly.

5. Bake for 20 minutes, or until the tops are golden brown. Test for doneness by lightly pressing on the center of the cookies: They should feel set. Let the cookies cool on the baking sheet, then store in an airtight container.

- -

GLUTEN FREE, NUT FREE *(replace almond flour with gluten-free flour; replace cashew butter with seed butter; omit cashews or substitute with pepitas)*, VEGAN, DAIRY FREE

irish breakfast oats

When I was 22, my husband and I spent a month backpacking through Europe. We did a week in Ireland, where we met my Irish cousins, tasted Guinness for the first time, and sang along loudly with musicians in the local pub. That trip connected me with my Irish roots, and I just couldn't get enough of it. So whenever I see McCann's Irish oatmeal at the grocery store, I just have to buy it to make this Irish treat. **SERVES 4**

4 cups water
¼ teaspoon sea salt
1 cup gluten-free steel-cut oats
1 tablespoon pure maple syrup
1 tablespoon almond butter

SUGGESTED TOPPINGS
1 ripe banana, sliced
½ cup sliced almonds
Dash of ground cinnamon

1. In a 4-quart saucepan, bring the water and salt to a boil. Add the oats and stir well. Reduce the heat to low and cook for 30 to 40 minutes, or until cooked through. The oats will be chewy, but they should not have any crunch.

2. Stir in the maple syrup and almond butter, then spoon the oatmeal into 4 bowls. If using any suggested toppings, add them now.

GLUTEN FREE, NUT FREE *(replace almond butter with sunflower butter)*, VEGAN, DAIRY FREE

rawkstar tip

To save time in the morning, soak the oats overnight in water and cook for 10 to 15 minutes in the morning. Or make a big batch at once and reheat individual servings throughout the week.

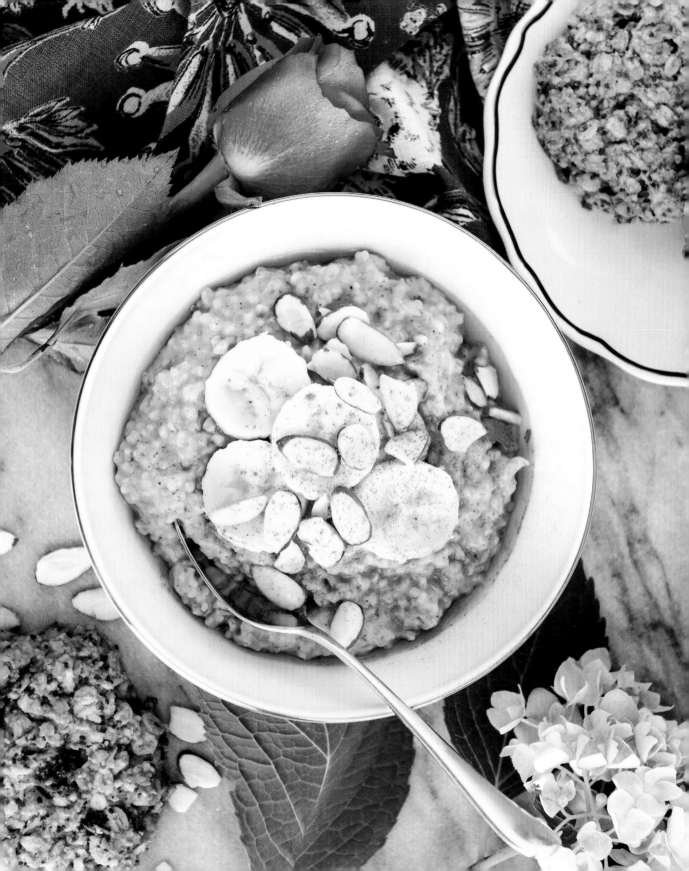

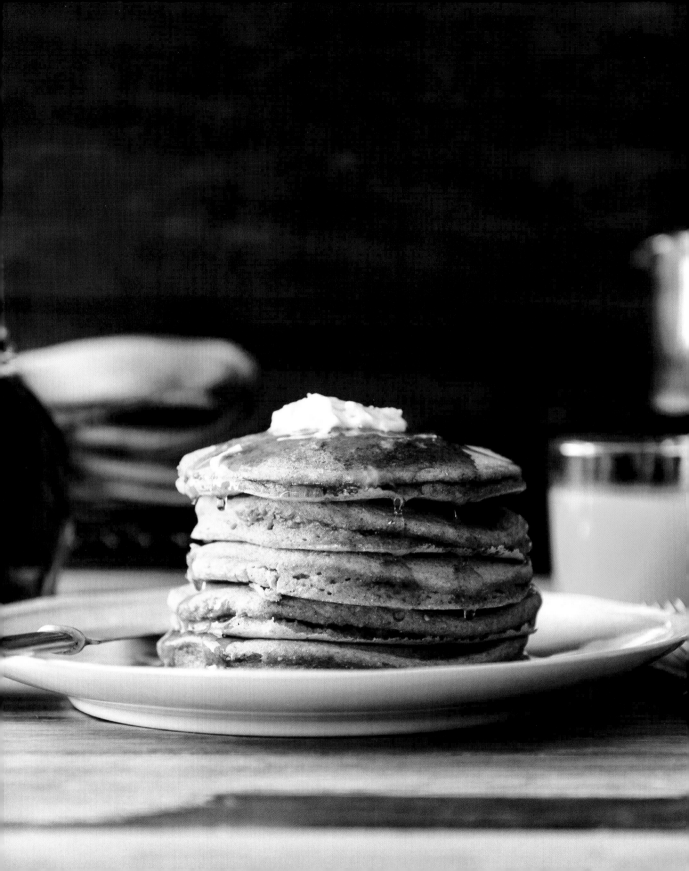

pumpkin spice pancakes

Confession: I have never been a fan of pumpkin pie—I actually remember gagging as a child when trying to eat a slice of it at Thanksgiving. After that, I always went for my Aunt Marci's apple pie. It wasn't until I tried a pumpkin-spiced latte that my love of pumpkin began—and resulted in smoothies, pancakes, and bread. This recipe is all about the pumpkin, which makes it extra-moist and flavorful and adds vital nutrients to a breakfast staple. SERVES 4

2 cups whole wheat flour
1 tablespoon baking powder
2 teaspoons pumpkin pie spice
½ teaspoon sea salt
2 cups unsweetened plain almond milk, plus more as needed
1 cup canned pure pumpkin puree

2 eggs, lightly beaten
2 tablespoons pure maple syrup
1 tablespoon organic virgin coconut oil, melted, plus more for cooking

SUGGESTED TOPPINGS
4 tablespoons pure maple syrup
1 teaspoon ground cinnamon

1. In a large mixing bowl, whisk together the flour, baking powder, spice blend, and salt.

2. In another large mixing bowl, whisk together the almond milk, pumpkin, eggs, maple syrup, and melted oil. Pour the pumpkin mixture into the flour mixture and stir until just combined. The mixture should have a few lumps. If the batter is too thick, thin it with a little more almond milk.

3. Heat a skillet over medium-high heat. Add a little oil and tilt the pan to spread the oil evenly. Ladle about ⅓ cup of the batter into the pan, working in batches as needed. Cook for 1 to 2 minutes, or until bubbles start forming on the top side and the edges begin to look dry and golden. Flip the pancakes carefully and cook for 1 to 2 minutes, or until cooked through. If using any suggested toppings, add them before serving.

GLUTEN FREE *(replace whole wheat flour with gluten-free all-purpose flour)*, NUT FREE *(replace almond milk with coconut milk)*, VEGAN *(replace eggs with "chia eggs": In a small bowl, stir together 2 tablespoons chia seeds and 6 tablespoons water; let stand for 10 minutes before adding to recipe)*, DAIRY FREE

sweet potato hash

I could eat this for breakfast every day of my life—it's that good. It reminds me of a diner in my hometown of Lancaster, California, called Crazy Otto's. I used to go there with my running ladies for the hash browns and omelets on Saturday mornings to celebrate our friendship. This recipe takes it up a level with kale, sweet potatoes, and lots of warming spices. It also makes a great dinner when you're running low on ideas or energy. Anyone else a fan of breakfast for dinner? **SERVES 2**

2 tablespoons organic virgin coconut oil
1 yellow onion, diced
Sea salt and ground black pepper
2 sweet potatoes, diced
3 garlic cloves, minced
2 teaspoons paprika

Pinch of ground red pepper (optional)
2 cups kale, stems removed and cut into
   thin ribbons

SUGGESTED TOPPINGS
2 eggs, fried in coconut oil
Red pepper flakes or hot sauce

1. Heat a large skillet over medium-high heat. Add the oil to the pan and let it warm for 30 to 60 seconds. Add the onion and sprinkle with a little salt. Cook, stirring frequently, until the onion starts to soften and turn golden on the edges.

2. Add the sweet potatoes and season to taste with salt and black pepper. Cook, turning frequently for even browning. When the sweet potatoes are almost cooked through, stir in the garlic, paprika, and red pepper, if using. Continue to cook, turning frequently, until the sweet potatoes are cooked through.

3. Add the kale and gently turn everything over to mix well. Cook for 1 to 2 minutes, or until the kale has wilted. Add more salt, black pepper, and red pepper to taste.

4. Divide between 2 plates and add the suggested toppings as desired.

GLUTEN FREE, NUT FREE, VEGAN *(skip the eggs)*, DAIRY FREE

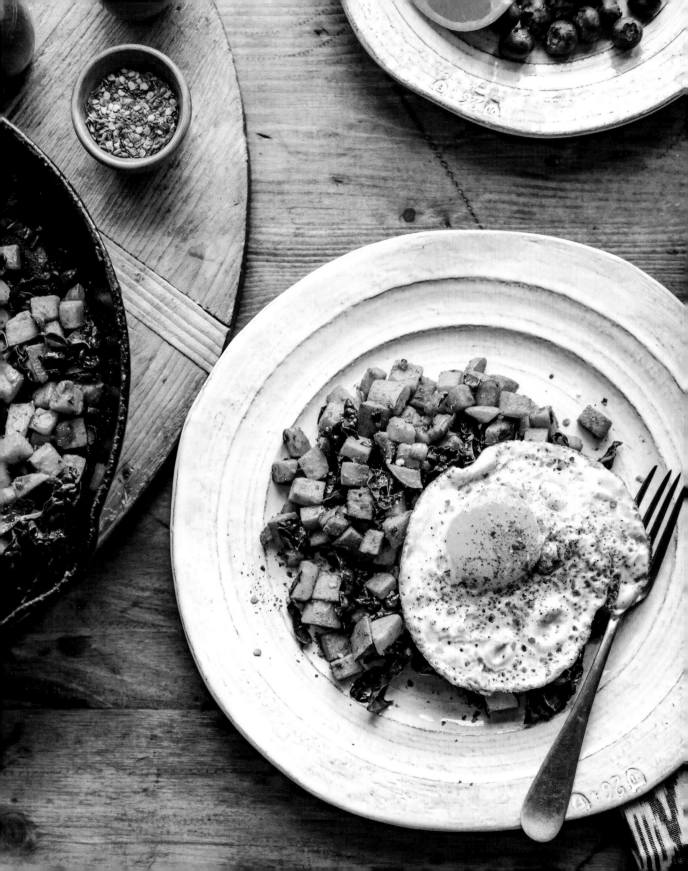

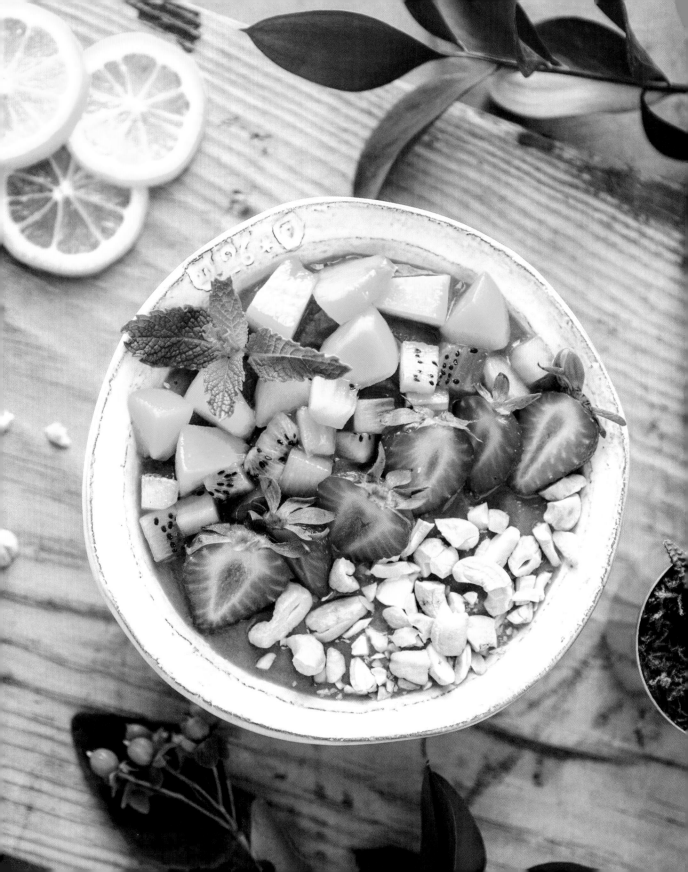

sunrise smoothie bowl

Every chance I get to take the kids fruit picking, I do it. It's so important that they understand where our food comes from and how beautiful nature is! This past summer, we found a local peach orchard and spent the afternoon filling up our baskets and our bellies. We ate just as much as we bought and left with happy tummies and dreams for what recipes we would make next. This smoothie bowl came from that day. **SERVES 2**

2 cups fresh spinach
½ cup water
1 orange, peeled and segmented
2 cups sliced peaches, preferably frozen
1 ripe banana, frozen
1 tablespoon fresh lemon juice

½ cup sliced strawberries
½ cup diced peaches
1 kiwifruit, diced
¼ cup raw cashews
4 fresh mint leaves, chopped

1. In a blender, puree the spinach, water, and orange until smooth. Add the sliced peaches and the banana and pulse a few times, then puree until the mixture is thick and smooth. You will need to stop the blender occasionally to scrape down the sides. Add a little extra water if needed. The texture should be thick and creamy like frozen yogurt.

2. Divide between 2 bowls and top each with half of the strawberries, diced peaches, kiwi, cashews, and mint. Serve immediately.

GLUTEN FREE, NUT FREE *(replace cashews with ¼ cup hemp hearts)*, VEGAN, DAIRY FREE

spicy sunrise sandwich

There's something very creative and adventurous about using hash browns as your bun—and I am all about that. Start your day with this breakfast sandwich that'll power you through with lots of energy and stamina thanks to the healthy fats and protein. Carpe diem! **SERVES 4**

FOR HASH BROWN BUNS
1 bag (20 ounces) shredded hash
  browns, thawed
½ yellow onion, finely minced
3 eggs
½ teaspoon sea salt
Ground black pepper
4 tablespoons avocado oil, divided

FOR SANDWICHES
1 cup fresh spinach
1 ripe avocado, sliced
4 eggs, fried in coconut oil
Coconut Sriracha Sauce, for serving
  (opposite)

1. *To make the buns:* Place the thawed hash browns in a clean dishtowel and squeeze any excess liquid from the potatoes. You want them fairly dry. Transfer the hash browns to a large mixing bowl. Add the onion, eggs, salt, and pepper to taste and stir until well combined. The mixture may seem too dry at first, but don't add extra eggs or liquid.

2. Heat a skillet over medium-low heat. (Cooking at a lower heat for a longer time allows the edges to get crispy and brown and the center to cook through properly. Don't rush by raising the heat or turning the patties too quickly, or the "buns" may fall apart.) Add 2 tablespoons of the oil to the pan and heat for 30 seconds. Working in batches, use an ice cream scoop or a ⅓-cup measuring cup to make 8 "buns" by scooping the hash brown mixture into the pan and gently pressing down to form flattened disks that are 3 to 4 inches in diameter. Cook for 5 to 6 minutes, then carefully flip the patties and cook for 3 to 4 minutes, or until golden brown and mildly crispy.

3. Transfer the "buns" to a plate lined with a clean dishtowel to drain off any excess oil. Keep warm until ready to assemble the sandwiches.

4. *To make the sandwiches:* Place ¼ cup spinach followed by one-quarter of the sliced avocado and 1 fried egg onto each of 4 buns. Drizzle with the Coconut Sriracha Sauce and top with another hash brown bun. Serve immediately.

GLUTEN FREE, NUT FREE *(replace almond butter with 1 tablespoon tahini in Coconut Sriracha Sauce)*, VEGAN *(remove eggs and turn "bun" into hash brown scramble; replace honey in sauce with pure maple syrup)*, DAIRY FREE

COCONUT SRIRACHA SAUCE MAKES ABOUT ¾ CUP

½ cup canned full-fat coconut milk

2 tablespoons Sriracha sauce

1 tablespoon almond butter

1 teaspoon tamari

1 teaspoon honey

½ teaspoon Dijon mustard

In a small bowl, whisk together the ingredients. Refrigerate until ready to use.

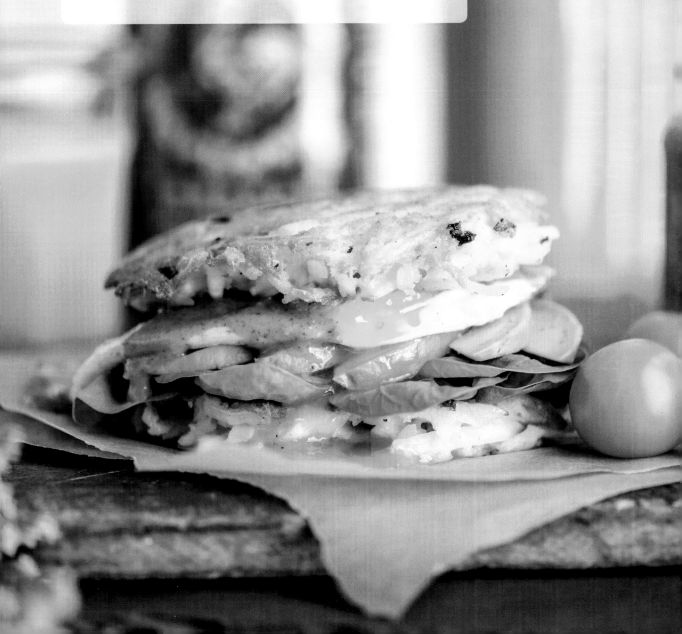

rawkstar parfait SERVES 2

⅓ cup fresh strawberries
⅓ cup fresh raspberries
⅓ cup fresh blueberries

2 cups unsweetened plain cashew
  yogurt
½ cup Pecan Granola (opposite)
2 teaspoons honey

In a small bowl, gently stir together the strawberries, raspberries, and blueberries. Into each jar or glass, layer, in this order: ½ cup of the yogurt, ¼ cup of the berries, 2 tablespoons of the granola, ½ cup of the yogurt, ¼ cup of the berries, 2 tablespoons of the granola. Top with a drizzle of honey.

GLUTEN FREE, NUT FREE *(replace cashew yogurt with coconut yogurt and modify granola recipe)*, VEGAN *(replace honey with maple syrup)*, DAIRY FREE

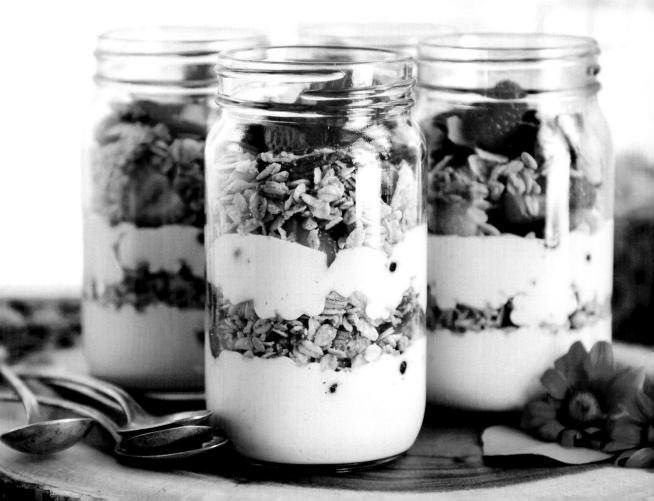

pecan granola

A few summers ago, my husband and I took a group of high school kids up to Georgia to cowork and live communally on a farm. It was a little hippy-ish, but we liked that. Every day, as sweat dripped down our backs, we picked blueberries and walked through pecan groves swatting flies. Ever since then, I have been in love with pecans and the regal trees they grow from. Whenever I bake this recipe, it brings me back to that summer in Georgia when we truly learned what it means to work for your food. **SERVES 8**

2 cups gluten-free rolled oats
1 cup unsweetened shredded coconut
1 cup pecans, roughly chopped
⅓ cup almond meal
½ cup pure maple syrup

¼ cup organic virgin coconut oil, melted
2 teaspoons pure vanilla extract
¼ teaspoon ground cinnamon
¼ teaspoon sea salt

1. Preheat the oven to 350°F. Line a rimmed baking sheet with parchment paper or a silicone baking mat.

2. In a large bowl, stir together the oats, coconut, pecans, and almond meal.

3. In a small bowl, stir together the maple syrup, oil, vanilla, cinnamon, and salt. Pour the maple mixture over the oats mixture and stir well to coat everything. Spread the mixture in an even layer on the prepared baking sheet.

4. Bake for 10 minutes, then stir, spread again in an even layer, and bake for 10 to 15 minutes, or until everything is golden and toasted.

5. Let cool completely. Transfer the cooled granola to an airtight container and store at room temperature.

GLUTEN FREE, NUT FREE (replace pecans with 1 cup pepitas and remove almond meal), VEGAN, DAIRY FREE

maple-walnut muffins

Grab and go is typically how breakfast happens at our house. We're either rushing off to school, church, baseball practice, or gymnastics competitions, or we're heading out to hit the trail for a run. It's rare for us to have a quiet, slow morning, and we've learned to create breakfasts that work for us. These muffins speak my love language because they can be made ahead and snagged on the way out the door. **MAKES 12 MUFFINS**

1 cup almond flour
1 cup gluten-free oat flour
2 tablespoons ground flaxseed
½ teaspoon ground cinnamon
2 teaspoons baking powder
½ teaspoon baking soda
½ teaspoon sea salt

½ cup pure maple syrup, at room temperature
¼ cup organic virgin coconut oil, melted
2 eggs, at room temperature
1 teaspoon pure vanilla extract
¾ cup grated apple (about 1 whole apple)
½ cup walnuts, chopped

1. Preheat the oven to 350°F. Line a standard muffin pan with paper liners or grease the cups very well.

2. In a large bowl, whisk together the almond flour, oat flour, flaxseed, cinnamon, baking powder, baking soda, and salt.

3. In a glass measuring cup or small mixing bowl, whisk together the maple syrup, oil, eggs, and vanilla.

4. Make a well in the center of the flour mixture. Pour the maple syrup mixture into the well. Stir until combined. Add the apple and walnuts and stir until combined.

5. Fill the muffin cups three-quarters full. (The batter does not rise while baking, so the cups will not overflow.) Bake for 20 to 25 minutes, or until the tops spring back when lightly pressed and a wooden pick inserted in the center of the muffins comes out almost clean. Allow to cool for 10 minutes before serving.

- -

GLUTEN FREE, NUT FREE *(replace almond flour with gluten-free all-purpose flour and remove the walnuts)*, VEGAN, DAIRY FREE

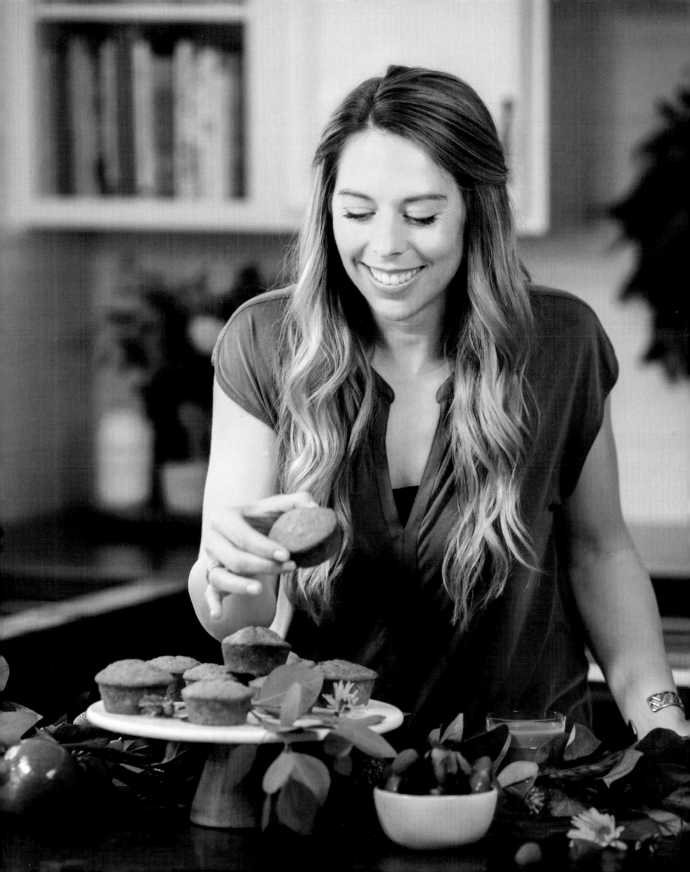

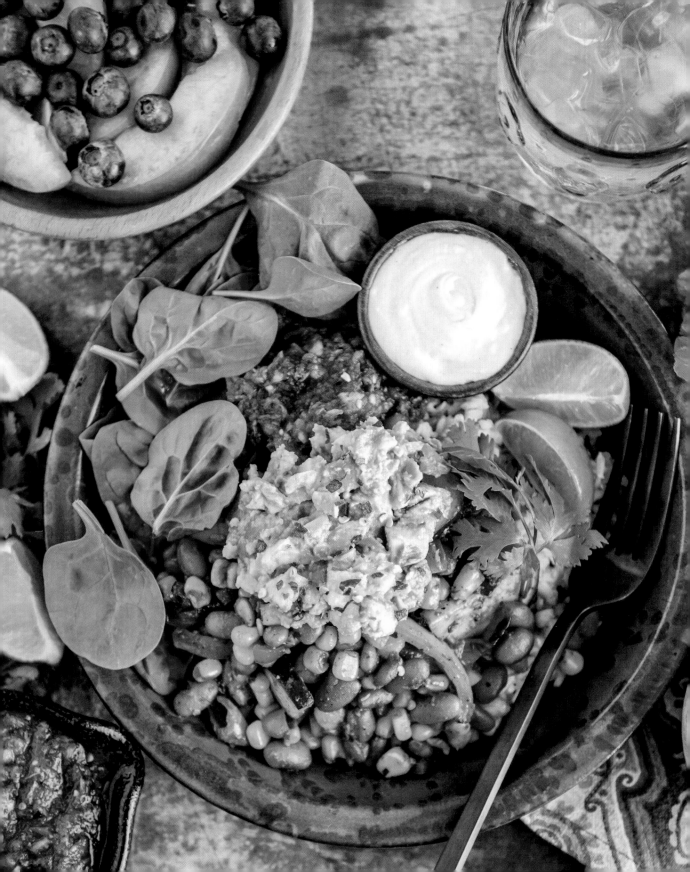

tex-mex breakfast bowl

Most of my weekends are filled with family activities, so I try to eat a good, hearty breakfast to kick-start the day. This breakfast bowl is how I start to fuel my day's adventures. **SERVES 4**

1 tablespoon avocado oil
1 yellow onion, cut into strips
1 orange bell pepper, cut into strips
1 zucchini, cut into ¼-inch pieces
1 jalapeño chile pepper, minced
3 garlic cloves, minced
2 teaspoons chili powder
1 teaspoon ground cumin
1 can (15 ounces) pinto beans, drained
and rinsed

1 cup organic corn kernels
Sea salt and ground black pepper
3 cups cooked brown rice, warmed
2 cups fresh spinach

SUGGESTED TOPPINGS
½ cup Legit Salsa (page 91)
4 tablespoons Cashew Cream (below)
1 ripe avocado, mashed
Pinch of red-pepper flakes
4 lime wedges

1. Heat a skillet over medium-high heat. Add the oil and warm for 30 seconds. Add the onion and bell pepper and cook for 3 minutes. Add the zucchini and cook for 5 minutes, or until just tender. Add the chile pepper and garlic and cook for 2 minutes. Stir in the chili powder, cumin, beans, and corn and cook until heated through. Season with salt and pepper.

2. Divide the cooked rice among 4 shallow bowls. Spoon the bean mixture on top, followed by the spinach. Top as desired, with a lime wedge on the side.

CASHEW CREAM MAKES ABOUT 1 CUP

1 cup raw cashews
4 tablespoons fresh lemon juice, divided

¼ cup water
Pinch of sea salt

1. Place the cashews in a medium bowl. Pour 2 tablespoons of the lemon juice over the top. Add enough water to cover by a few inches. Let soak 2 hours, then drain and rinse well.

2. In a food processor or blender, combine the cashews, ¼ cup water, salt, and the remaining 2 tablespoons lemon juice. Puree until smooth and creamy. Stop to scrape down the sides, as needed, and add a little more water if the mixture is too thick. Transfer to an airtight container. It will keep 4 days in the refrigerator or up to a month in the freezer.

GLUTEN FREE, NUT FREE *(without Cashew Cream)*, VEGAN, DAIRY FREE

cinnamon coffee cake

The first thing I ever remember baking was coffee cake when I was 8 years old. I remember getting out the Bisquick box and following the recipe on the side all by myself. When the cake came out of the oven and smelled so good, I ate the entire thing on my own. This recipe is a healthier twist on my original creation—yet it still satisfies my taste buds. **SERVES 9**

FOR STREUSEL AND TOPPING
½ cup unbleached all-purpose flour
½ cup coconut sugar
2 teaspoons ground cinnamon
½ teaspoon ground nutmeg
¼ teaspoon sea salt
6 tablespoons organic virgin coconut oil, at room temperature, plus more for greasing the pan
1 cup pecans, chopped

FOR CAKE
2½ cups unbleached all-purpose flour
1 tablespoon baking powder
½ teaspoon sea salt
½ cup organic virgin coconut oil, at room temperature
½ cup pure maple syrup
3 eggs, at room temperature
2 teaspoons pure vanilla extract
1 cup unsweetened plain almond milk, at room temperature

1. Preheat the oven to 350°F. Grease a 9 × 9-inch baking pan.

2. *To make the streusel and topping:* In a medium bowl, combine the flour, sugar, cinnamon, nutmeg, and salt. Add the oil and stir until combined. Set aside.

3. *To make the cake:* In a large mixing bowl, whisk together the flour, baking powder, and salt. In another bowl, whisk together the oil, syrup, eggs, and vanilla until smooth. Whisk in the almond milk. Make a well in the center of the flour mixture and add the almond milk mixture all at once. Sit until just combined.

4. Spread half of the cake batter in the prepared pan. Drop half of the streusel mixture evenly over the batter. Place the remaining batter over the streusel layer. Using the tip of a knife, gently swirl to create a marbled effect.

5. Add the pecans to the bowl with the remaining streusel. Stir to combine and sprinkle evenly over the batter in the pan.

6. Bake for 40 to 45 minutes, or until a wooden pick inserted in the center of the cake comes out clean and the top is golden. Let the cake cool slightly before serving.

GLUTEN FREE *(replace flour with gluten-free all-purpose flour)*, NUT FREE *(replace 1 cup pecans with 1 cup coconut flakes; replace 1 cup almond milk with 1 cup unsweetened plain coconut milk)*, VEGAN *(replace 3 eggs with 2 ripe bananas, mashed)*, DAIRY FREE

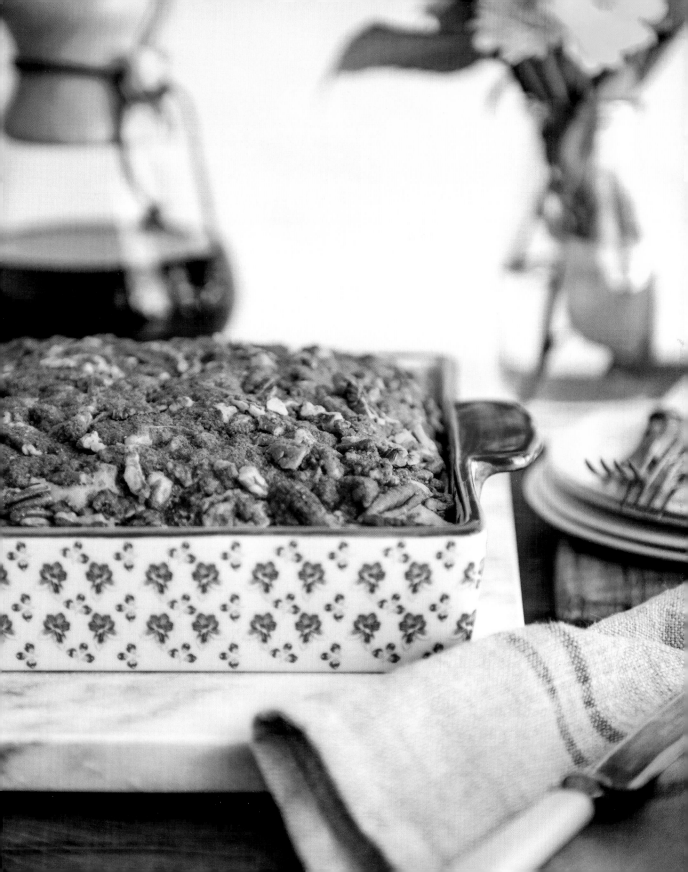

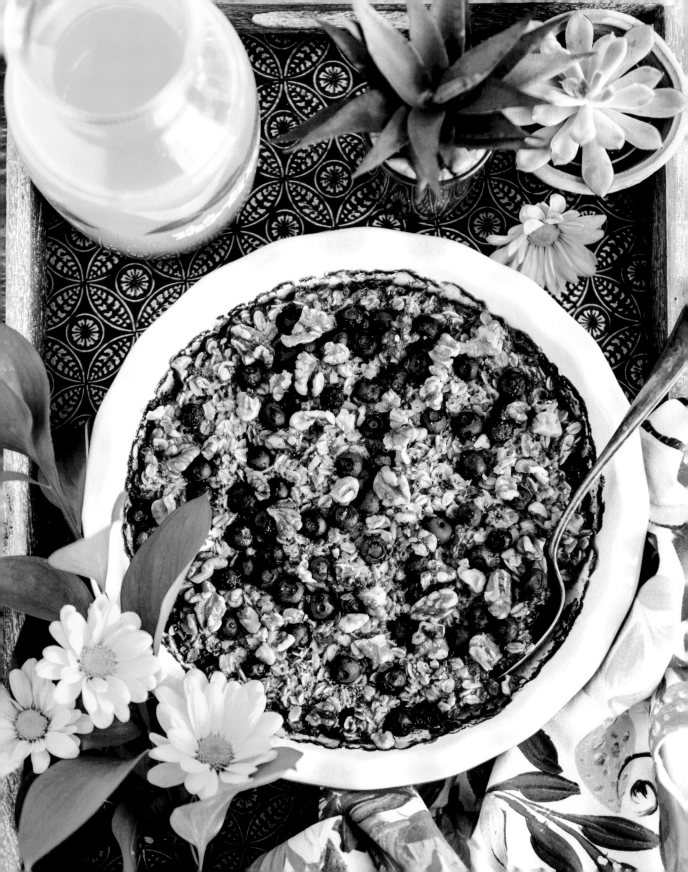

fairy-tale porridge

This porridge is swirling with spices and natural sweeteners that make it "just right" for even the pickiest of eaters. It's packed with many plant-powered superfoods, too—chia seeds, walnuts, and coconut oil, all containing healthy fats to help with skin hydration and digestive issues. **SERVES 4**

2 cups unsweetened plain almond milk
2 tablespoons chia seeds
1½ cups gluten-free rolled oats
2 tablespoons pure maple syrup
2 tablespoons organic virgin coconut oil, melted

1 teaspoon ground cinnamon
½ teaspoon pure vanilla extract
¼ teaspoon sea salt
1 ripe banana
1 cup blueberries
½ cup chopped walnuts

1. Preheat the oven to 350°F.

2. In a small bowl, combine the almond milk and chia seeds and whisk well. Let sit for 5 minutes, or until the seeds absorb some of the milk.

3. In a medium bowl, combine the rolled oats, maple syrup, oil, cinnamon, vanilla, and salt. Whisk in the chia mixture.

4. Slice the banana and distribute in an even layer on the bottom of a 9 × 5-inch baking dish. Top with ½ cup of the blueberries. Pour the oats mixture over the top. Sprinkle the remaining berries and the chopped walnuts over the top.

5. Bake for 35 to 40 minutes, or until the center is set and the top is golden brown. Serve warm.

GLUTEN FREE, NUT FREE *(replace almond milk with unsweetened plain coconut milk; remove walnuts)*, VEGAN, DAIRY FREE

power protein bowl

I have been obsessed with veggie bowls for a few years now. This breakfast bowl is a take on a classic dinner one, yet it is kicked up a notch with the insanely addictive pesto that I slather over every single bite. It's truly the best pesto I've ever had. **SERVES 2**

1 cup dry quinoa

2 cups vegetable stock

1 cup baby kale

1 teaspoon extra-virgin olive oil

2 hard-boiled eggs, sliced

1 ripe avocado, sliced

4 tablespoons Sun-Dried Tomato Pesto (below)

1. If the quinoa is not prerinsed (check the package), place it in a fine-mesh sieve and rinse well with cool water to remove the bitter saponins on the quinoa. Drain well.

2. In a large saucepan, combine the quinoa and stock. Bring to a boil, then reduce the heat to low and cover the pan. Cook for 15 to 20 minutes, or until the quinoa is cooked through. Let stand for 5 to 10 minutes.

3. In a medium bowl, combine the kale and oil and massage for 2 to 3 minutes, or until the kale softens.

4. To serve, divide the quinoa into 2 shallow bowls. Top each with half of the kale, 1 sliced egg, half of the avocado, and 2 tablespoons of the pesto. Serve immediately.

SUN-DRIED TOMATO PESTO MAKES 1½ CUPS

½ cup raw almonds

1 cup oil-packed sun-dried tomatoes, undrained

½ cup fresh basil

1 small shallot

1 garlic clove

¼ teaspoon sea salt

Extra-virgin olive oil, if needed

Place the almonds in a food processor or blender and pulse until finely chopped. Add the tomatoes, basil, shallot, garlic, and salt and pulse until everything is finely chopped but not completely pureed. If the machine is having trouble processing, add a little olive oil. Taste and add more salt, if needed. Transfer to a jar with a tight-fitting lid. Store in the refrigerator for up to 1 week or freeze for several months.

GLUTEN FREE, VEGAN *(replace eggs with 1½ cups canned chickpeas)*, DAIRY FREE

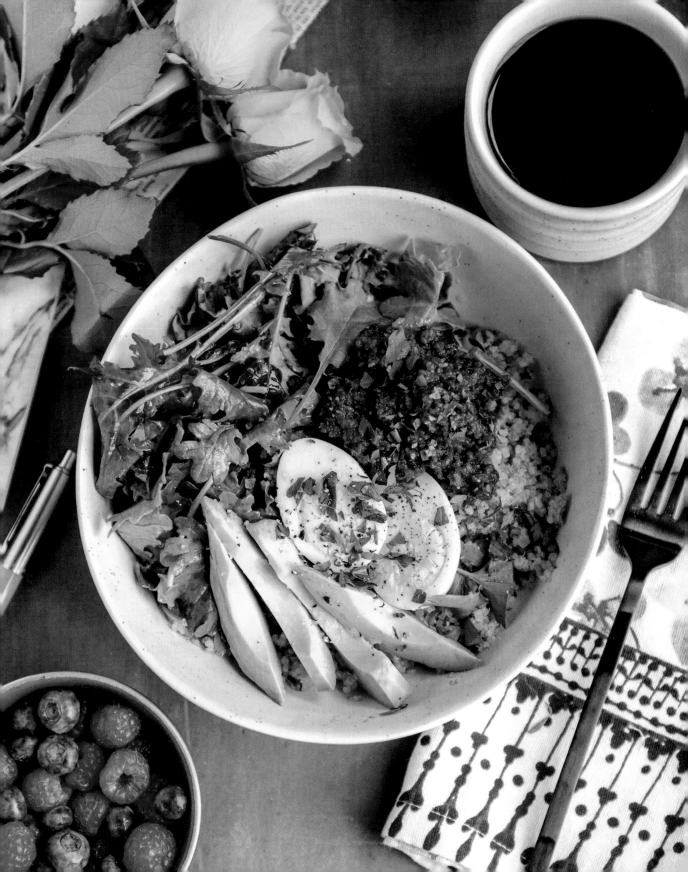

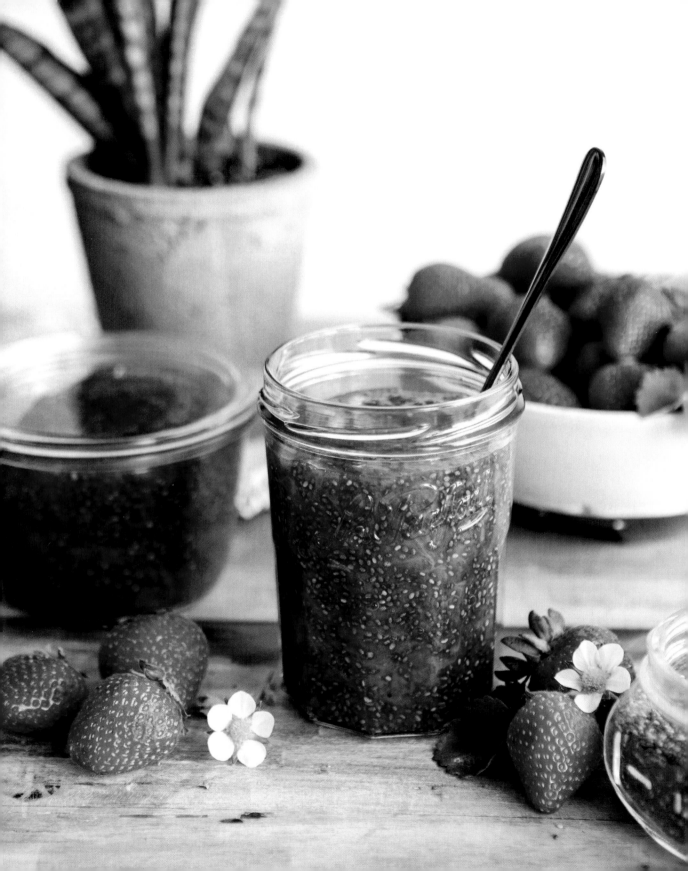

strawberry chia jam

When Jackson was first diagnosed with a corn sensitivity, I felt like my life was over. Pretty much every packaged food in America contains corn in some form or another—including jam. I started making my own jam using the fresh Florida strawberries we picked in spring. This recipe uses chia seeds to thicken the mixture into jam instead of pectin, which often contains dextrose—a sweetener made from corn. **MAKES 2 CUPS**

1 pound fresh strawberries, hulled
   and halved
¼ cup water
¼ cup pure maple syrup

3 tablespoons fresh lemon juice
   (from 1 lemon)
2–3 tablespoons chia seeds
1 teaspoon pure vanilla extract

1. In a medium saucepan, combine the strawberries, water, maple syrup, and lemon juice. Bring to a simmer and cook for 15 to 20 minutes, or until the fruit softens and releases its natural juices. Mash the mixture well.

2. Stir in the chia seeds. Start with 2 tablespoons, especially if the strawberry mixture is pretty thick. Different fruits have different moisture contents and may require more or fewer chia seeds for the jam to set. Let the jam cool completely on the counter. Stir again and add more chia seeds if the jam is too runny or thin. Stir in the vanilla. Transfer to small jars with tight-fitting lids.

3. Store in the fridge for 7 to 10 days or freeze for up to several months. If storing in the freezer, be sure to leave ½-inch headspace in the jar to allow for expansion.

GLUTEN FREE, NUT FREE, VEGAN, DAIRY FREE

almond butter and jam muffins

I adapted this recipe from Lindsey's fabulous blog, *Café Johnsonia*. The jam on the inside was such a fun idea and tastes *soooooo* good! My whole family adores these muffins, but I definitely love them the most. These muffins bring back childhood peanut butter and jelly sandwiches in a sophisticated and more nutritious way. **MAKES 12 MUFFINS**

⅓ cup almond butter
¼ cup organic virgin coconut oil, at room temperature
½ cup pure maple syrup
2 eggs
1 teaspoon pure vanilla extract
¾ cup unbleached all-purpose flour
¾ cup whole wheat flour

1½ teaspoons baking powder
¼ teaspoon baking soda
¼ teaspoon sea salt
¼ teaspoon ground cinnamon
½ cup unsweetened plain almond milk
6 tablespoons thick jam, preferably all-fruit and naturally sweetened

1. Preheat the oven to 400°F. Line a 12-cup muffin pan with paper liners.

2. In a large bowl, and using an electric mixer on high speed, beat the almond butter and oil until creamy. Add the maple syrup and beat until well combined. Add the eggs and vanilla and continue beating until creamy.

3. In a separate bowl, whisk together the flour, baking powder, baking soda, salt, and cinnamon. Add one-third of the flour mixture to the creamed mixture and beat on low speed just until combined. Add half of the almond milk and beat again. Add another third of the flour mixture, followed by the rest of the almond milk, and ending with the remaining flour mixture. Continue mixing just until the batter comes together. Do not overmix.

4. Using a small ice cream scoop or spoon, fill the muffin cups one-quarter full. Use the tip of a spoon to push the batter to cover the entire bottom and a little up the sides. Place 1 rounded teaspoon of jam in each muffin cup, trying to center it as much as possible. Top the jam with the remaining batter, making sure it covers the jam.

5. Bake for 15 to 20 minutes, or until the tops are golden brown and spring back when gently pressed. Let cool in the pan for 10 minutes, then remove and serve.

GLUTEN FREE *(replace flour with 1½ cups gluten-free all-purpose flour)*, VEGAN *(replace eggs with ½ cup applesauce)*, DAIRY FREE

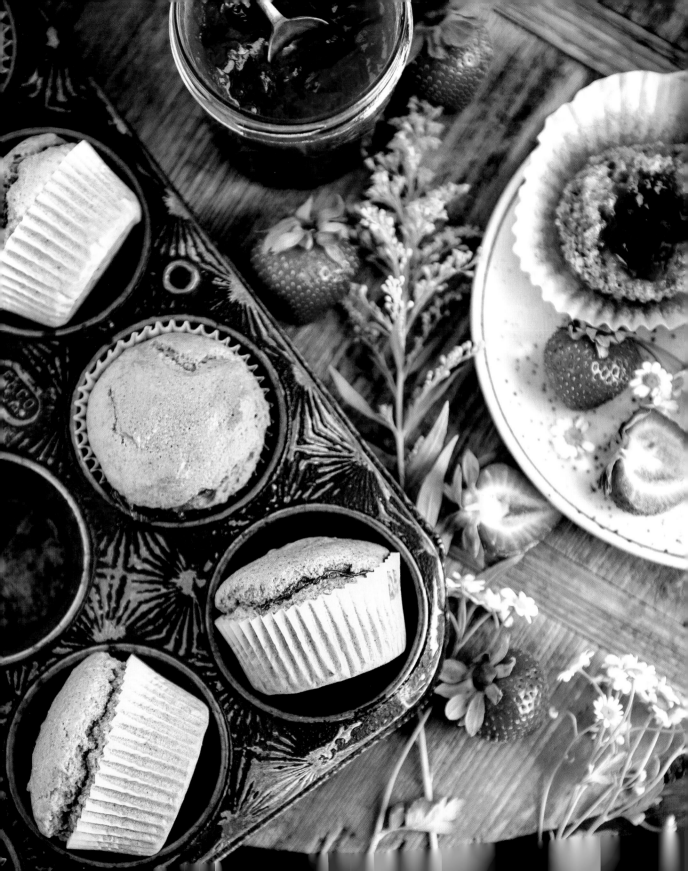

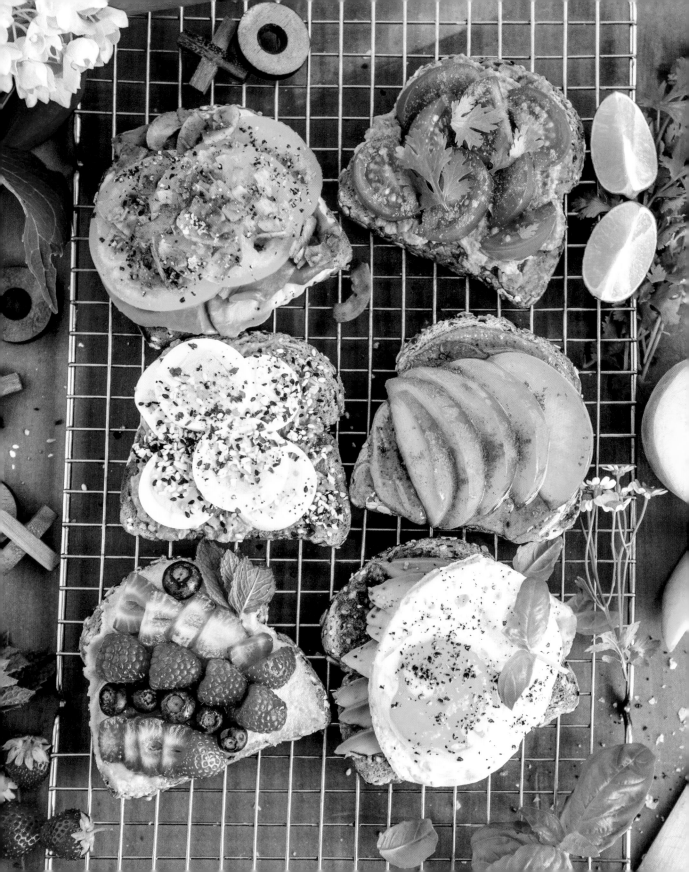

breakfast toast—six ways

I am not one to eat the same breakfast every day. I need change or I lose interest—and you won't want to be around me if I haven't had breakfast (it's dangerous!). These variations on the classic toast of my childhood get me excited about all the variety breakfast can contain. I hope they help you out, too, and maybe inspire some toast variations of your own!

EACH VARIATION SERVES 1

Choose your variation, toast the bread lightly, layer on your toppings, and enjoy!

CBLT

1 slice whole wheat or gluten-free bread
1 tablespoon Cashew-Garlic Aioli
   (page 132)
¼ ripe avocado, mashed
1 leaf tender lettuce (such as butter lettuce)
½ ripe tomato, sliced
2 tablespoons Coconut Bacon (page 80)
Pinch of coarsely ground black pepper
Pinch of sea salt

SPICY AND LOADED

1 slice whole wheat or gluten-free bread
¼ ripe avocado, mashed
1 hard-boiled egg
Pinch of crushed red-pepper flakes
Everything Bagel Sprinkle (page 81)

BERRIES 'N' CREAM

1 slice whole wheat or gluten-free bread
1 tablespoon Cashew Cream (page 67)
½ cup berries, sliced if needed
Fresh mint, for garnish
Drizzle of honey

MEXICAN TOAST-ADA

1 slice whole wheat or gluten-free bread
2 tablespoons refried beans or smashed black
   or pinto beans
¼ ripe avocado, sliced
½ ripe tomato, sliced
⅛ teaspoon fresh lime juice
Pinch of sea salt
Pinch of ground cumin
2 teaspoons fresh cilantro, chopped

PEACHY

1 slice whole wheat or gluten-free bread
1 tablespoon almond butter
½ peach, pitted and thinly sliced
Drizzle of honey
Pinch of ground cinnamon

TUSCAN SUNSHINE

1 slice whole wheat or gluten-free bread
2 tablespoons Sun-Dried Tomato Pesto
   (page 72)
¼ ripe avocado, sliced
1 fried egg

COCONUT BACON MAKES 2 CUPS

2 tablespoons tamari
2 tablespoons pure maple syrup
1 teaspoon liquid smoke
2 cups unsweetened wide-flaked
   coconut strips

½ teaspoon paprika
¼ teaspoon ground black pepper
¼ teaspoon sea salt

1. Preheat the oven to 350°F. Line a baking sheet with parchment paper.

2. In a small bowl, stir together the tamari or soy sauce, maple syrup, and liquid smoke.

3. Place the coconut in a bowl and pour the tamari mixture over the top. Toss gently to coat. Sprinkle the paprika and black pepper over the top and toss gently again.

4. Spread the coconut mixture evenly on the prepared baking sheet. Bake for 10 to 15 minutes, or until golden. Let cool completely. Store in an airtight container in the refrigerator for up to 1 week.

EVERYTHING BAGEL SPRINKLE MAKES ½ CUP

3 tablespoons sesame seeds
1 tablespoon poppy seeds
1 tablespoon dried minced
   onion

1 tablespoon dried minced
   garlic
1 teaspoon sea salt

In a jar with a lid, combine the sesame seeds, poppy seeds,
onion, garlic, and salt. Attach the lid and store the jar in a
cool, dry place. Keeps for several months.

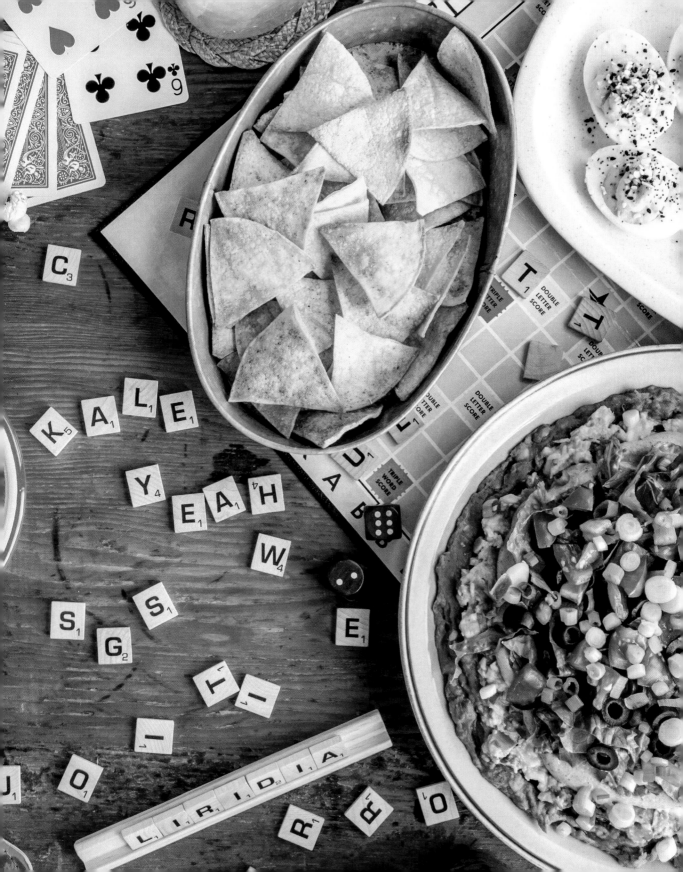

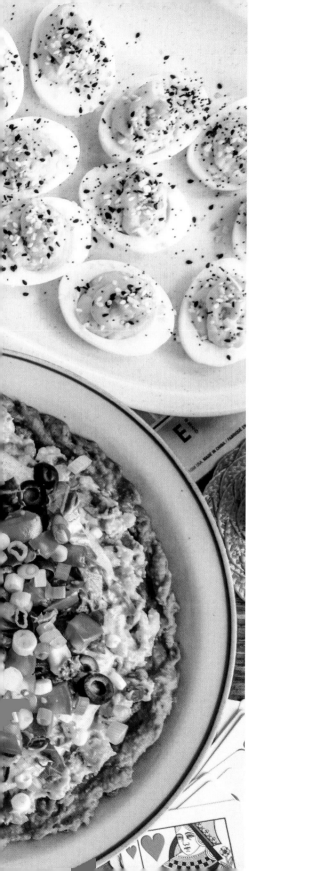

snacks

great smoky almonds

Almonds are a great snack raw, but some days I need a little flavor oomph to motivate me to eat another almond. Maple syrup and liquid smoke do the trick! I like to bring healthy snacks along on our annual road trip up to Raleigh, North Carolina, to see my brother and his family. This recipe has come along for the 10-hour ride, which is where it got its name. **SERVES 4**

1 tablespoon avocado oil
2 teaspoons liquid smoke
1 teaspoon pure maple syrup

2 cups raw almonds
½ teaspoon sea salt
¼ teaspoon garlic powder

1. Preheat the oven to 350°F. Line a baking sheet with parchment paper.

2. In a medium mixing bowl, combine the oil, liquid smoke, and maple syrup. Add the almonds and stir until well coated. Sprinkle the salt and garlic powder over the almonds and stir again.

3. Spread the almonds on the prepared baking sheet. Bake for 10 to 12 minutes, or until the nuts are nicely toasted. Let cool completely before storing in an airtight container.

GLUTEN FREE, VEGAN, DAIRY FREE

rawkstar tip

Any nuts can be used in place of the almonds, if desired. Baking time may be slightly different, so check for doneness after about 8 minutes.

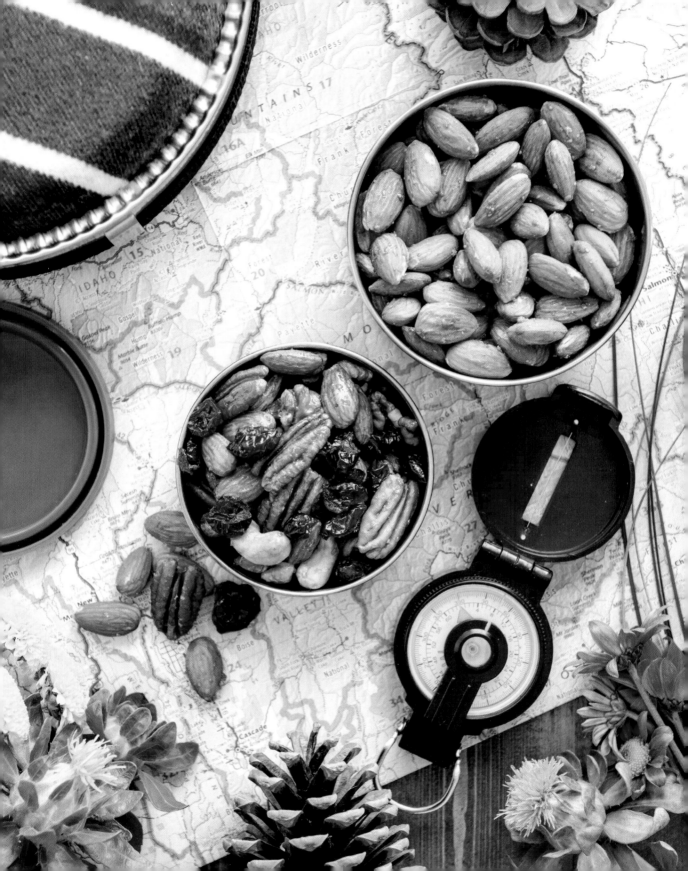

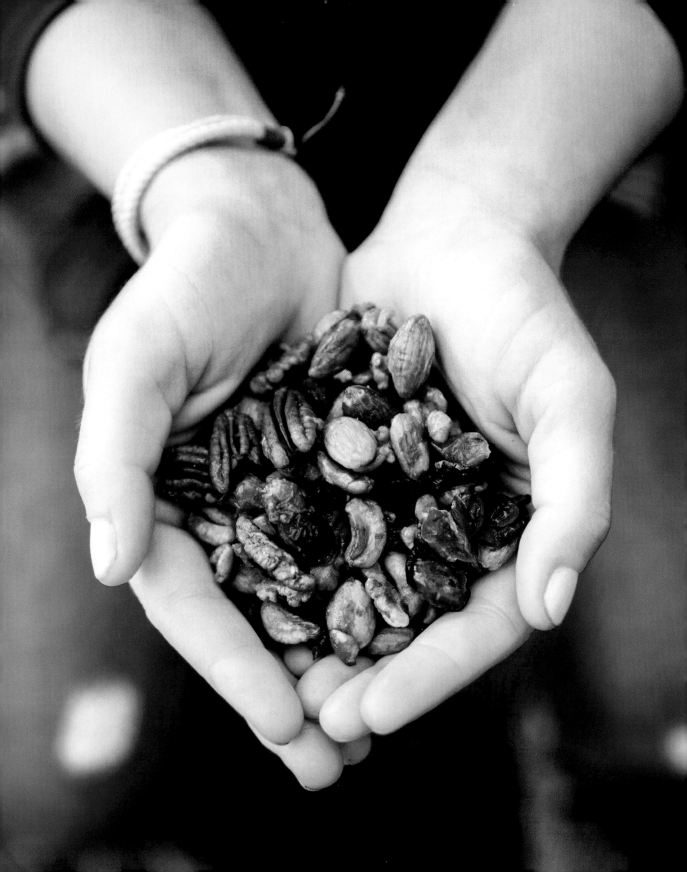

honey nut trail mix

Trail mix is a versatile snack to keep in your work drawer, to store in the glovebox of your car to grab while waiting in the after-school pickup line, or to bring along on a long run or hike. Packed with protein and salty sweetness, this mix will fuel you in no time! **SERVES 8**

2 tablespoons honey, warmed slightly
1 tablespoon organic virgin coconut oil, melted
1½ teaspoons pure vanilla extract
½ teaspoon pure almond extract
½ teaspoon sea salt

1 cup raw walnuts
1 cup raw cashews
1 cup raw almonds
1 cup raw pecans
2 cups dried cranberries

1. Preheat the oven to 350°F. Line a baking sheet with parchment paper.

2. In large bowl, stir together the honey, oil, vanilla, almond extract, and salt. Add the nuts and stir until they are evenly coated with the honey mixture.

3. Spread the coated nuts on the prepared baking sheet. Bake for 15 minutes, stir, and bake for 5 to 10 minutes longer, or until the nuts are toasted and the honey has caramelized.

4. Once the nuts have cooled completely, add the cranberries and stir well. Transfer to an airtight container.

GLUTEN FREE, VEGAN *(replace 2 tablespoons honey with 2 tablespoons maple syrup)*, DAIRY FREE

rawstar tip

I try to use raw nuts as much as possible to retain more nutrients, yet feel free to swap out with roasted nuts depending on what you can find.

sweet potato chips

My husband, Ryan, bought me a mandoline a few months ago, and I have since gone to town with this handy slicer. I make these sweet potato chips on a weekly basis because they are such a simple, quick (and filling!) bite when paired with Holy Guacamole (below). **SERVES 6**

¾ cup organic virgin coconut oil, or more as needed

3 sweet potatoes, cut into ⅛-inch slices
Sea salt

1. Heat the oil in large skillet over medium-high heat. Add the sweet potatoes in batches and cook for 5 to 10 minutes, flipping the slices occasionally, until crispy. Remove any chips that have cooked more quickly than the others, placing the finished chips on a paper towel–lined plate to absorb excess oil.

2. Repeat the process until all the slices are cooked. Season with sea salt and enjoy while warm.

GLUTEN FREE, NUT FREE, VEGAN, DAIRY FREE

holy guacamole **SERVES 8**

4 ripe avocados, halved and pitted
1 ripe tomato, diced and seeds removed
½ cup fresh cilantro, roughly chopped
1 jalapeño chile pepper, minced, seeds and ribs removed

2 garlic cloves, minced
2 tablespoons fresh lime juice
½ teaspoon sea salt

1. In a medium bowl, mash the avocados well with a fork. Stir in the tomato, cilantro, chile pepper, garlic, lime juice, and salt.

2. Serve immediately, or cover tightly and refrigerate until ready to eat. It will keep several days refrigerated. To prevent browning, press plastic wrap or waxed paper directly on the surface of the guacamole and/or place an avocado pit in the center.

GLUTEN FREE, NUT FREE, VEGAN, DAIRY FREE

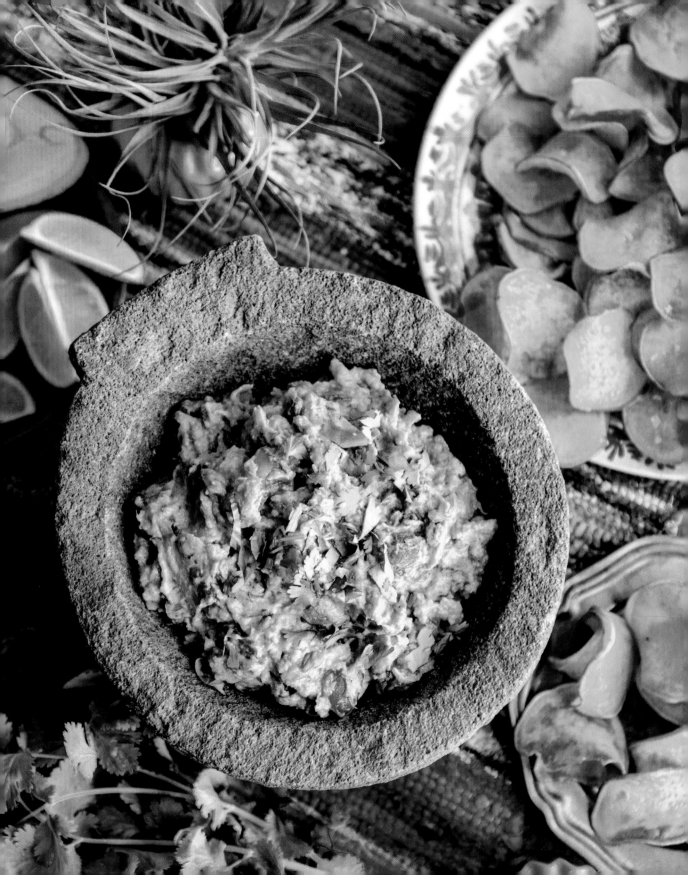

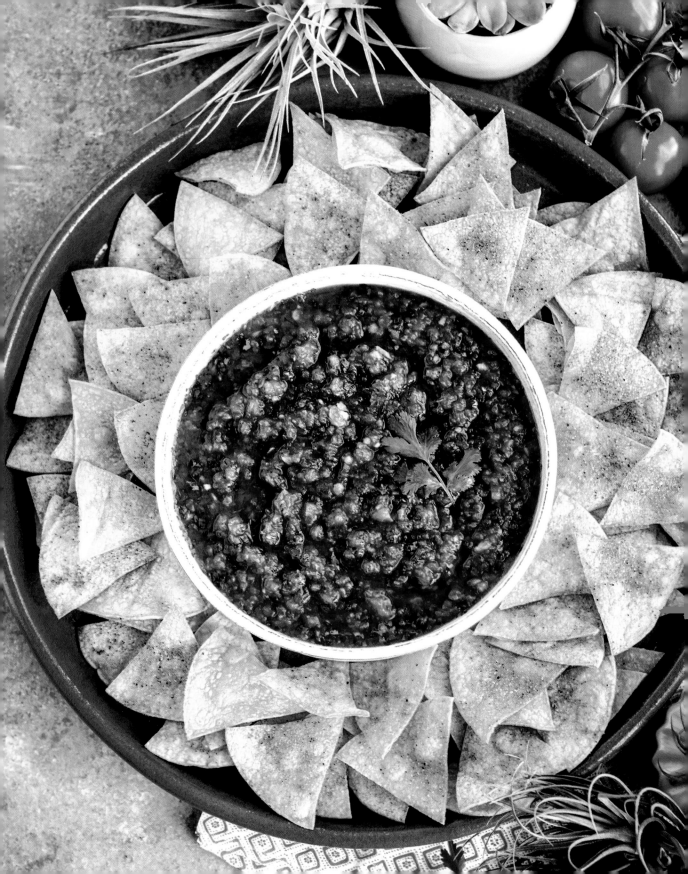

baked tortilla chips

Try these homemade chips if you're looking to eat as fresh as possible. Cooking time varies based on your oven, so pay attention to get the perfect chip. **SERVES 6**

12 organic corn tortillas
¼ teaspoon chili powder
¼ teaspoon ground cumin
¼ teaspoon garlic powder

¼ teaspoon paprika
1 teaspoon organic virgin coconut oil, melted
Sea salt

1. Preheat the oven to 425°F. Line 2 baking sheets with parchment paper.

2. Cut each tortilla into 6 wedges, then arrange the wedges in an even layer on the prepared baking sheets. Bake for 10 minutes.

3. Remove from the oven and very lightly brush one side of the chips with the oil. (Too much oil and the chips will be chewy.) Sprinkle evenly with the spices and salt. Return the pans to the oven and bake for 5 to 8 minutes, or until golden.

GLUTEN FREE, NUT FREE, VEGAN, DAIRY FREE

legit salsa

When we moved to Florida, I missed L.A.'s amazing chips and salsa. My friend Lindsey fixed that yearning for me when she shared the most amazing version right here. **MAKES 5 CUPS**

2 jalapeño chile peppers, diced
1 yellow onion, quartered
1 small bunch fresh cilantro, leaves and tender stems
2 garlic cloves, halved

1 can (28 ounces) diced tomatoes, undrained
¼ cup fresh lime juice
1 teaspoon sea salt

In a blender, combine all the ingredients and pulse until the desired texture is reached. Taste and add more salt, if needed. Store in an airtight container in the refrigerator for up to 1 week.

GLUTEN FREE, NUT FREE, VEGAN, DAIRY FREE

emerald green gem

Jackson and Clare love their green smoothies as much as I do . . . especially when we use tropical fruits. This recipe, a family favorite, is easy to blend ahead and freeze in mason jars. Pack them in a cooler and allow them to defrost naturally on your next adventure. **SERVES 1**

1 cup fresh spinach	½ banana, peeled
½ cup water	¼ avocado, peeled
1 orange, peeled	½ cup frozen peaches

1. In a high-powered blender, mix the spinach, water, and orange until smooth and juice-like. Add the banana, avocado, and peaches, and mix again.

2. Serve over ice, if desired.

GLUTEN FREE, NUT FREE, VEGAN, DAIRY FREE

road trippin' with green smoothies

Cruising on the interstate as a family is in my DNA. When I was little, my parents would find the best airfare deal to somewhere in the United States, fly us all to that destination, and rent a car to road trip it for a few weeks. I learned so much about our beautiful nation. From bustling cities and historic battlegrounds to forests and waterfalls—we saw it all.

Now I do the same with my family and love every minute of it. Small-town tourist attractions, local coffee shops, national parks, charming main streets, and wide open spaces. On the road, discovering and learning, is where I get most lit up.

Since feeling good is super important to me, and eating well is a huge part of that, I've learned to take control of my health while on the road. We bring a cooler, a blender, cups, and straws—it's just part of my family's road trip packing routine. We blend our smoothies in the morning at the hotel, motel, or campground and sip them down for breakfast on the road. I usually blend extra and pour it into mason jars to store in the cooler for an afternoon snack. Each night, I'll rinse the cups in the hotel sink (or bathtub) and start fresh again the next day.

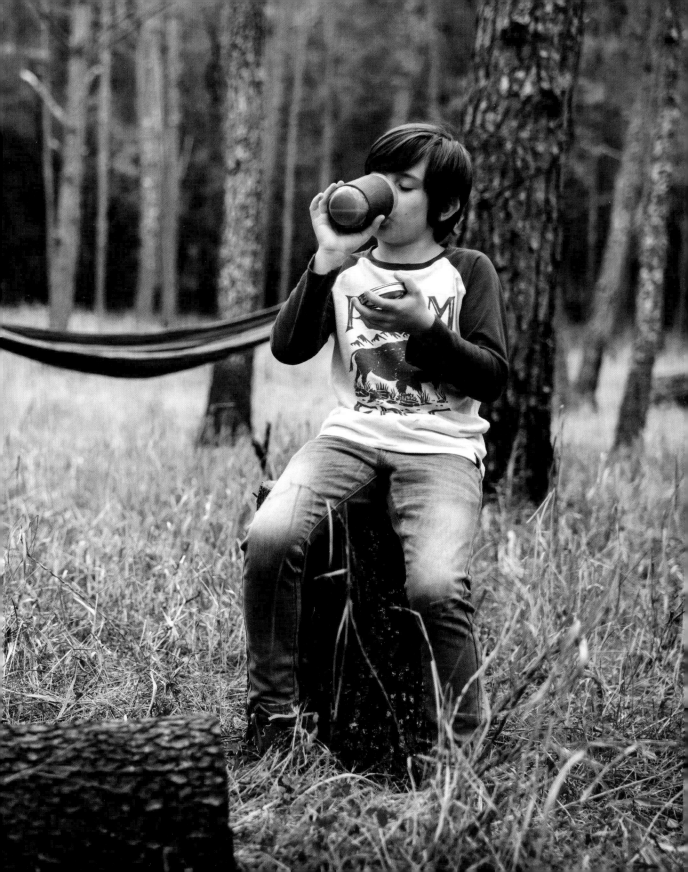

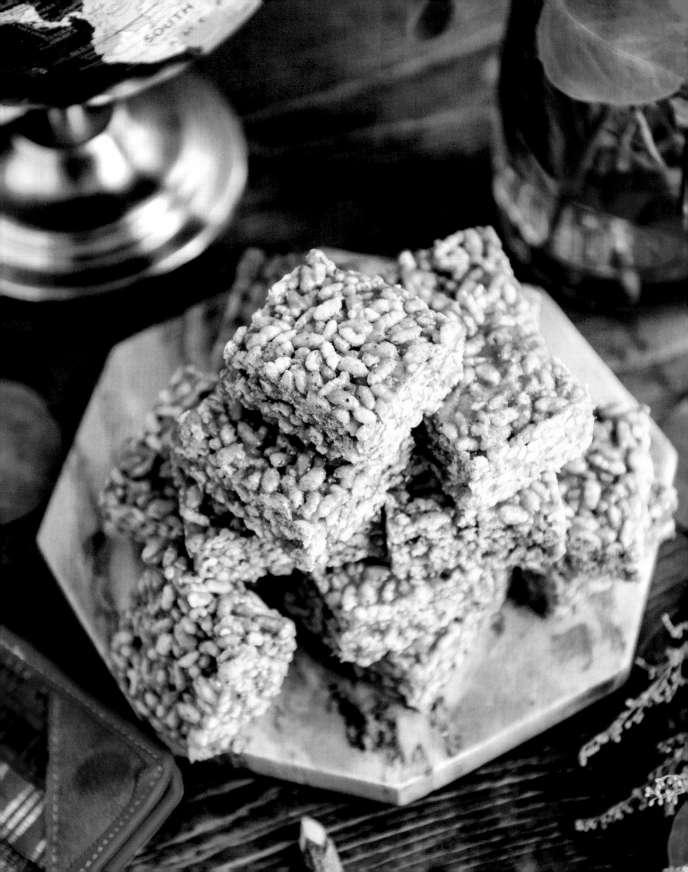

almond butter crisps

There's a restaurant in Tampa called Fresh Kitchen that rawks my world! They have amazing veggie bowls, and right before the register where you pay, they dangle almond butter treats in front of your face. I can never say no, and I never regret buying them either. They are amazing! This is my own version of those bars, and I think they turned out pretty dang good.

MAKES 16 SQUARES

1 cup brown rice syrup
2 tablespoons organic virgin coconut oil, plus more for greasing the pan
2 teaspoons pure vanilla extract

½ teaspoon sea salt
1 cup creamy almond butter
2 teaspoons ground cinnamon
7 cups crisp brown rice cereal

1. Line a 13 × 9-inch baking pan with parchment paper.

2. In a medium saucepan over medium-high heat, combine the rice syrup, oil, vanilla, and salt. Bring to a rolling boil. Boil for 1 minute, then remove from the heat. Stir in the almond butter and cinnamon.

3. Place the cereal in a large mixing bowl. Pour the almond butter mixture over the cereal and stir until well coated. Transfer the mixture to the prepared pan. Using oiled hands, press the mixture evenly into the pan. Let cool completely before cutting into squares.

GLUTEN FREE, NUT FREE *(replace almond butter with sunflower butter)*, VEGAN, DAIRY FREE

cacao crush smoothie

For years, I struggled with finding a plant-based protein powder that I enjoyed in smoothies. Eventually, I attempted to make my own using 100 percent organic, pure ingredients. I'm obsessed with how it turned out. The end result is a protein-packed powder that makes you feel as great as it tastes. **SERVES 1**

1½ cups unsweetened almond milk
½ cup frozen cauliflower
¼ avocado, peeled

1 serving Daily Blends cacao powder
½ teaspoon ground cinnamon
½ teaspoon pure vanilla extract

1. In a high-powered blender, combine the almond milk, cauliflower, avocado, Daily Blends cacao powder, cinnamon, and vanilla until smooth and creamy.

2. Serve immediately over a glass of ice.

GLUTEN FREE, VEGAN, DAIRY FREE

rawkstar tip

If you don't have my Daily Blends protein powder (http://sgs.to/powder), feel free to swap with 1 tablespoon raw cacao powder and 1 teaspoon honey to get a similar taste.

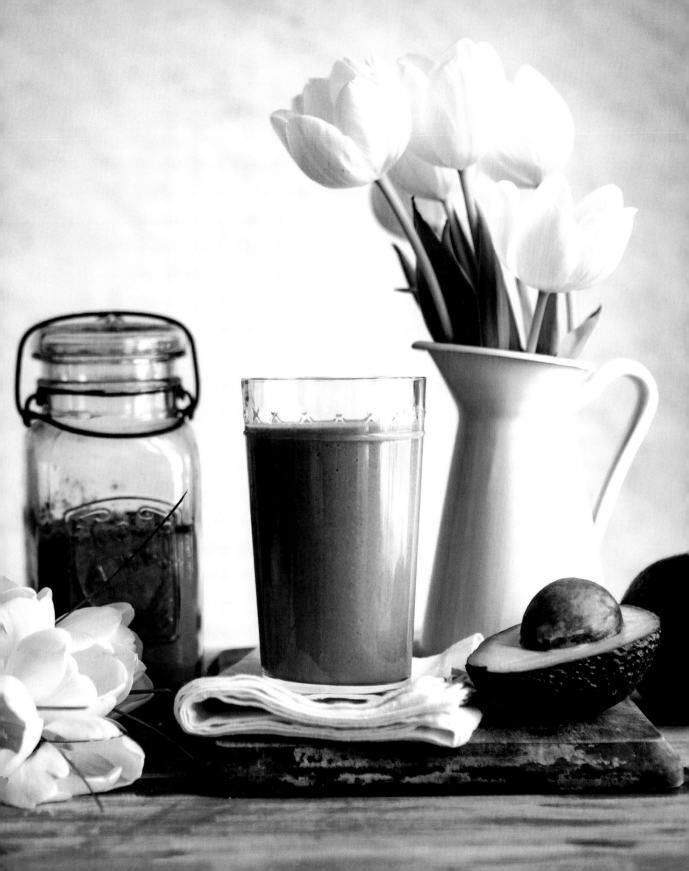

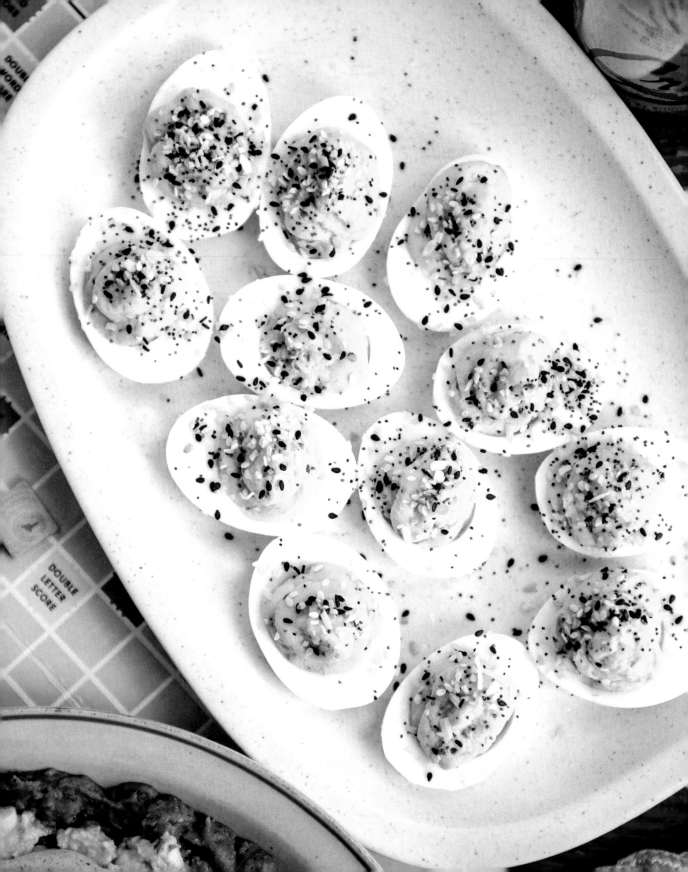

hansard farm deviled eggs

It wasn't until we moved to Brooksville, Florida, that I ever thought of having a farm. Yet the idea wasn't too farfetched for our small country town—so we went with it. Now we have seven hens and a duck that lay eggs daily and follow us around the yard. Deviled eggs were a tradition in my home growing up, but over the years I fell out of love with mayonnaise. This recipe uses hummus as a mayonnaise replacement, making it more flavorful and boosting the protein content. **MAKES 12 EGGS**

6 hard-boiled eggs, peeled and halved
8 tablespoons Simple Hummus
   (page 100)
2 tablespoons finely diced pickles

2 teaspoons yellow mustard
Sea salt and ground black pepper
Pinch of paprika per egg

1. Remove the egg yolks from the whites. Place the yolks in a medium mixing bowl and mash with a fork. Stir in the hummus, pickles, mustard, and a pinch of salt and pepper.

2. Place the egg white halves on a serving plate. Spoon the hummus mixture into the whites. Sprinkle with the paprika, then refrigerate, covered, until ready to serve.

VARIATION

Guac Deviled Eggs: Substitute Holy Guacamole (page 88) for the hummus and omit the mustard and pickles.

GLUTEN FREE, NUT FREE, DAIRY FREE

simple hummus

Yes, I am that girl who will eat carrot sticks just so I can eat the hummus. I love hummus so much! This recipe is a staple in our home. It has just the right amount of seasoning to motivate you to make another batch the second the container is empty. **MAKES ABOUT 2 CUPS**

1 can (15 ounces) chickpeas, drained and rinsed
¼ cup extra-virgin olive oil, plus more for drizzling
3 tablespoons fresh lemon juice (from 1 lemon)

½ cup tahini
3 garlic cloves
1 teaspoon ground cumin
½ teaspoon sea salt
Dash of paprika

1. In a food processor or blender, pulse the chickpeas until chopped. Add ¼ cup oil, the lemon juice, tahini, garlic, cumin, and salt and process or blend until smooth. Stop to scrape down the sides as needed.

2. Transfer the hummus to a bowl, then drizzle with oil and throw on a dash of paprika.

VARIATIONS

ROASTED RED PEPPER HUMMUS: Add ½ roasted red pepper (jarred or fresh), 1 teaspoon chili powder, and 1 teaspoon paprika.

PESTO HUMMUS: Add ¼ cup pesto.

SUN-DRIED TOMATO HUMMUS: Add ½ cup softened sun-dried tomatoes plus 1 teaspoon dried basil.

GLUTEN FREE, NUT FREE, VEGAN, DAIRY FREE

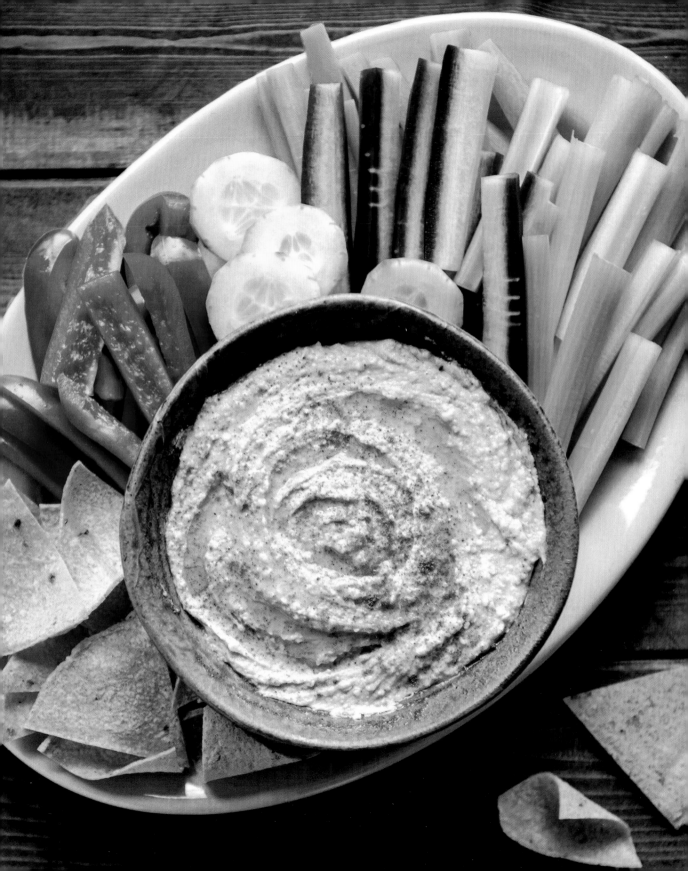

rawkstar tip

Swap the popcorn with roasted cauliflower florets for a low-carb, delicious treat.

cool ranch popcorn

This recipe embodies my entire childhood in a nutshell—yet without the artificial ingredients I have no clue how to pronounce or spell. Popcorn is high in fiber and pairs well with coconut oil, a healthy fat that holds up to higher heats. **SERVES 8**

2 tablespoons organic virgin coconut oil
½ cup organic popcorn kernels

1–2 tablespoons Cool Ranch Sprinkle (below)

1. Heat a 6-quart, heavy-duty pot (with tight-fitting lid) over medium-high heat. Add the oil and 1 corn kernel, and let the oil melt and get very hot. Once the kernel pops, add the rest of the kernels and put on the lid. As the kernels start to pop, gently shake the pan so the popcorn doesn't burn on the bottom.

2. When the popping slows, turn off the heat and let the last few kernels finish popping. Immediately transfer the popcorn to a large serving bowl.

3. While the popcorn is piping hot, spread 1 to 2 tablespoons of the ranch sprinkle evenly over the popcorn. Toss gently. Serve warm.

COOL RANCH SPRINKLE MAKES ¼ CUP

¼ cup nutritional yeast (if flaked, place in a blender to finely grind)
1 teaspoon dried dillweed
½ teaspoon paprika

½ teaspoon garlic powder
½ teaspoon onion
½ teaspoon sea salt
¼ teaspoon black pepper

In a small jar, combine the nutritional yeast, dillweed, paprika, garlic powder, onion, salt, and pepper. Attach the lid and shake to combine. Store in an airtight container in a cool, dry place.

GLUTEN FREE, NUT FREE, VEGAN, DAIRY FREE

vegan queso

As much as I love queso at my favorite Mexican restaurant, Pancho's Villa in San Antonio, Florida, it doesn't always love me back. The dairy and processed cheese do some strange things to my belly. (I'll stop there.) This vegan queso is the next best thing, and it keeps my body thriving all day. Infused with warming spices and a hearty texture, it's making tastebuds and bellies all over the world very happy.   **MAKES ABOUT 1 CUP**

1 cup raw cashews
3 tablespoons lemon juice (from 1 lemon), divided
¼ cup nutritional yeast
2 tablespoons chili powder
1 tablespoon tamari
1 teaspoon ground cumin

1 jalapeño chile pepper, ribs and seeds removed
1 garlic clove
Sea salt and ground black pepper
1–4 tablespoons water

FOR SERVING
Baked Tortilla Chips (page 91)

1. Place the cashews in a medium bowl and pour 2 tablespoons of the lemon juice over them. Add enough water to cover by a few inches. Let soak for 2 hours, then drain and rinse well.

2. In a high-powered blender, combine the cashews, nutritional yeast, chili powder, tamari, cumin, jalapeño, garlic, the remaining 1 tablespoon lemon juice, and salt and black pepper to taste. Puree until smooth, stopping to scrape down the sides as needed. Add 1 tablespoon of water at a time, as needed, to create a smooth sauce that is thick enough for dipping. Taste and add more salt, if needed.

3. Transfer to a bowl and serve with tortilla chips.

VARIATION

CHILI CON QUESO DIP: Stir in 1 can (15 ounces) black beans, drained, after you've pureed the dip.

GLUTEN FREE, VEGAN, DAIRY FREE

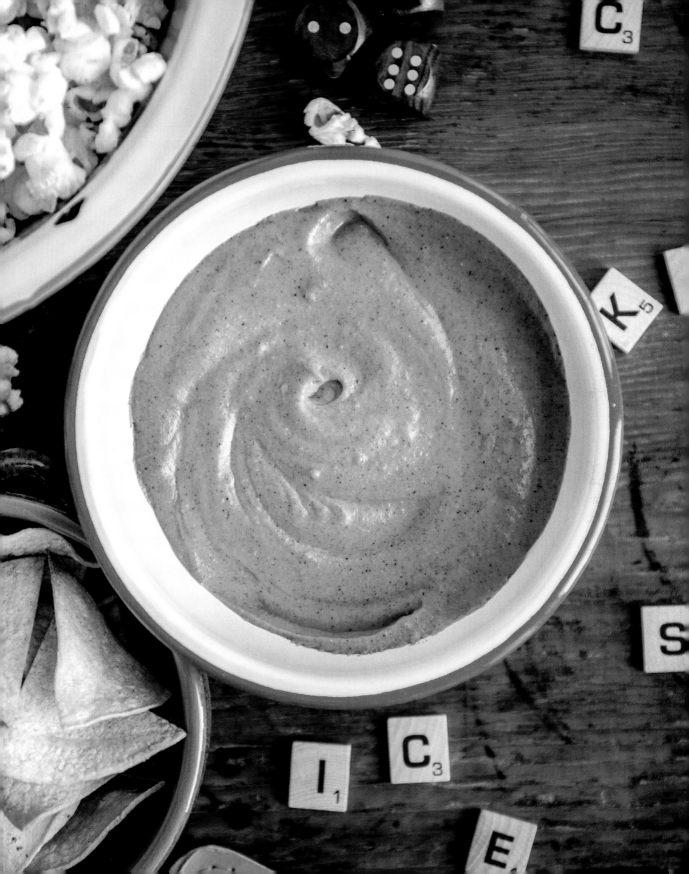

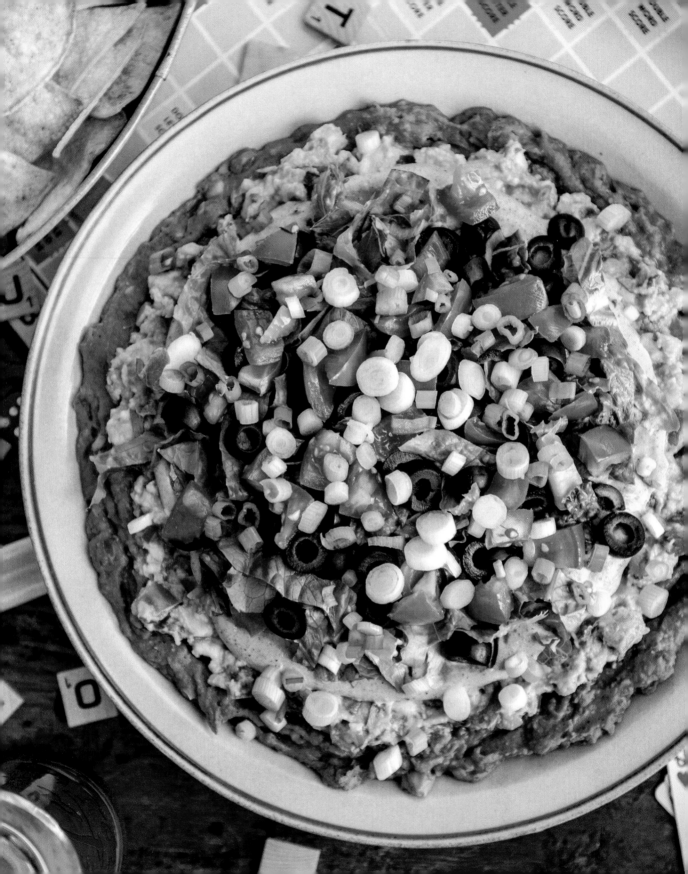

seven-layer dip

I could eat Mexican food for every meal of the day and never get tired of it. That is a fact. It may have started when my mom began making this dip as a Thanksgiving Day tradition when we were little. I've adjusted the recipe to use Cashew Cream instead of shredded Cheddar cheese, and it is delish! **SERVES 6–8**

1½ cups Loaded Frijoles (page 164)
1 cup Holy Guacamole (page 88)
1 cup Cashew Cream (page 67)
1 tablespoon taco seasoning or Simple Taco Seasoning (below)
2 cups shredded romaine lettuce

1 ripe tomato, seeded and diced
½ cup black olives, sliced
½ cup thinly sliced scallions

FOR SERVING
Baked Tortilla Chips (page 91)

1. On a large shallow platter, spread the *frijoles* (beans) in an even layer. Spoon the guacamole on top, then carefully spread it to cover the beans as best as possible.

2. In a small bowl, mix together the cashew cream and taco seasoning. Spread on top of the guacamole layer. (If the cream is thin, it may be easier to drizzle it.)

3. Top the cashew cream layer with the lettuce, followed by the tomato, olives, and scallions. Cover and refrigerate until ready to serve with tortilla chips.

SIMPLE TACO SEASONING

6 tablespoons chili powder
2 tablespoons ground cumin
4 teaspoons sea salt

4 teaspoons paprika
1 teaspoon ground red pepper (optional)

In an 8-ounce mason jar with lid, combine all the ingredients. Attach the lid and shake well. Store in a cool, dry place.

GLUTEN FREE, NUT FREE *(omit the cashew cream)*, VEGAN, DAIRY FREE

maple granola bars

When you need to go the extra mile, granola bars are your BFF. I grew up on Nature's Valley bars thanks to my dad, but I wanted to make my own version using my favorite plant-based ingredients. Now this, my friend, is a rawkstar granola bar. **MAKES 8 BARS**

1½ cups gluten-free rolled oats
½ cup almond flour
½ cup sliced almonds
½ cup pure maple syrup
½ cup raisins
¼ cup almond butter

2 tablespoons chia seeds
1 tablespoon organic virgin coconut oil, melted
1 teaspoon pure vanilla extract
½ teaspoon ground cinnamon
¼ teaspoon sea salt
Pinch of ground nutmeg

1. Preheat the oven to 325°F. Grease an 8 × 8-inch baking pan and line the bottom with parchment paper.

2. In a large bowl, combine the oats, almond flour, almonds, maple syrup, raisins, almond butter, chia seeds, oil, vanilla, cinnamon, salt, and nutmeg. Press the mixture into the prepared pan. Bake for 25 to 30 minutes, or until lightly golden on the edges. Let cool completely in the pan.

3. Cut into 8 rectangles. They will keep for about 1 week if wrapped well and stored in a cool place.

GLUTEN FREE, NUT FREE *(remove almonds, increase oats to 2 cups, and replace almond butter with sunflower butter)*, VEGAN, DAIRY FREE

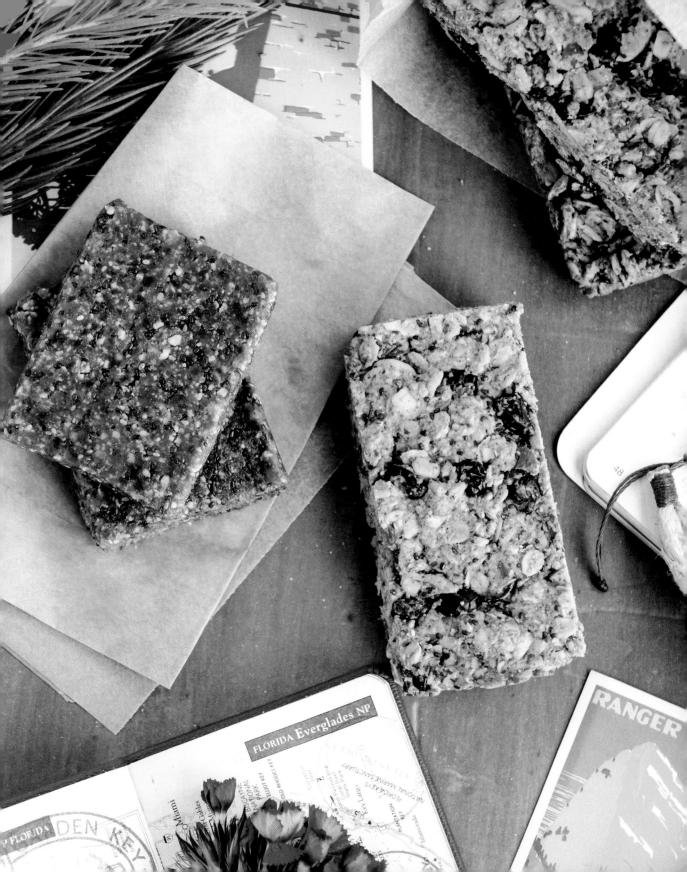

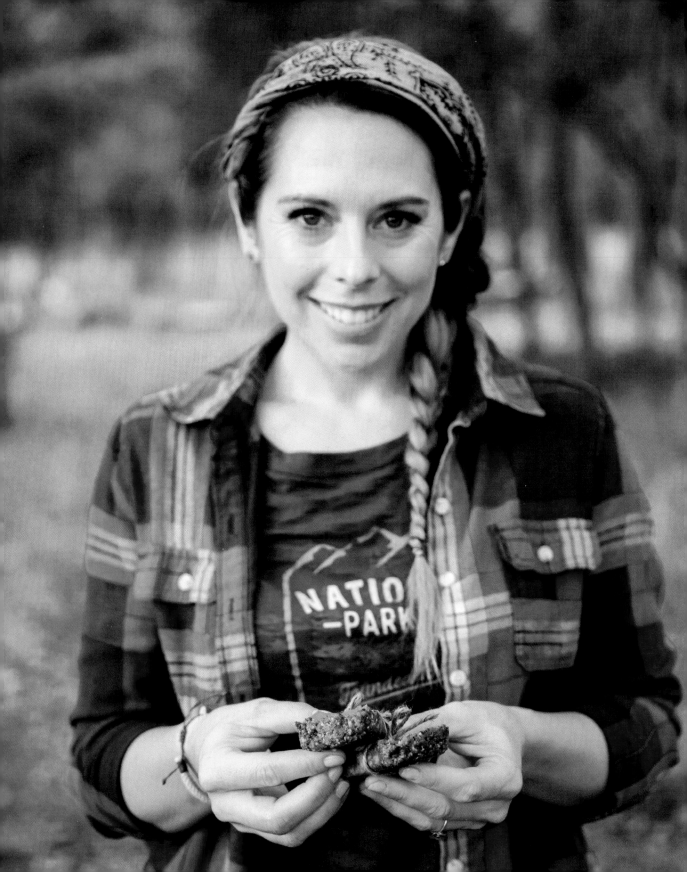

adventure bars

Next time you're heading out on a grand adventure, bake these bars. They're loaded with protein, natural sugars, and healthy fats thanks to the cashews and hemp hearts—and they have the most amazing chew factor going on thanks to the antioxidant-rich dried fruits. If you want your bars bite-size, cut them into 16 squares instead of 8 bars. **MAKES 8 BARS**

1 cup raw cashews
½ cup unsweetened shredded coconut
1 cup medjool dates, pitted
½ cup dried apricots

½ cup dried tart cherries
4 tablespoons chia seeds
4 tablespoons hemp hearts
½ cup creamy almond butter

1. In a food processor fitted with the chopping blade, combine the cashews and coconut and pulse until finely chopped. Transfer to a bowl.

2. Place the dates in the food processor. Pulse a few times, then process the dates until they have turned into a paste. Add the apricots and cherries and pulse a few times. Return the cashew mixture to the fruit, along with the chia seeds, hemp hearts, and almond butter. Process until the ingredients are well combined—neither too dry nor too sticky—and hold together nicely when pressed. If the mixture is too crumbly, add a little more almond butter or a tiny bit of water and process again.

3. Lay a piece of parchment paper on a clean, flat surface and turn the mixture out onto it. Press the mixture together and form into an 8-inch square that is a little thicker than ¼ inch. Place in the fridge or freezer to firm up before cutting into 8 bars.

4. Wrap the bars individually in parchment paper. They will keep for several weeks in the fridge or several months in the freezer.

GLUTEN FREE, VEGAN, DAIRY FREE

spa pops

On a hot summer day, it's important to nourish and hydrate your body so that you can run around, having fun and thriving. Oftentimes, we mistake dehydration for exhaustion or hunger. These refreshing pops make it super easy to keep yourself fueled and hydrated as the temperature goes up. **SERVES 6**

3 cups seeded and cubed ripe watermelon

1 cup peeled, seeded, and diced cucumber

2 tablespoons fresh lime juice

2 tablespoons fresh mint leaves

Honey (optional)

1. In a blender, combine the watermelon, cucumber, lime juice, and mint and puree until very smooth. Taste the mixture and add honey if you want a sweeter treat.

2. Pour the mixture into ice-pop molds and freeze overnight, or until firm.

GLUTEN FREE, NUT FREE, VEGAN *(omit the honey)*, DAIRY FREE

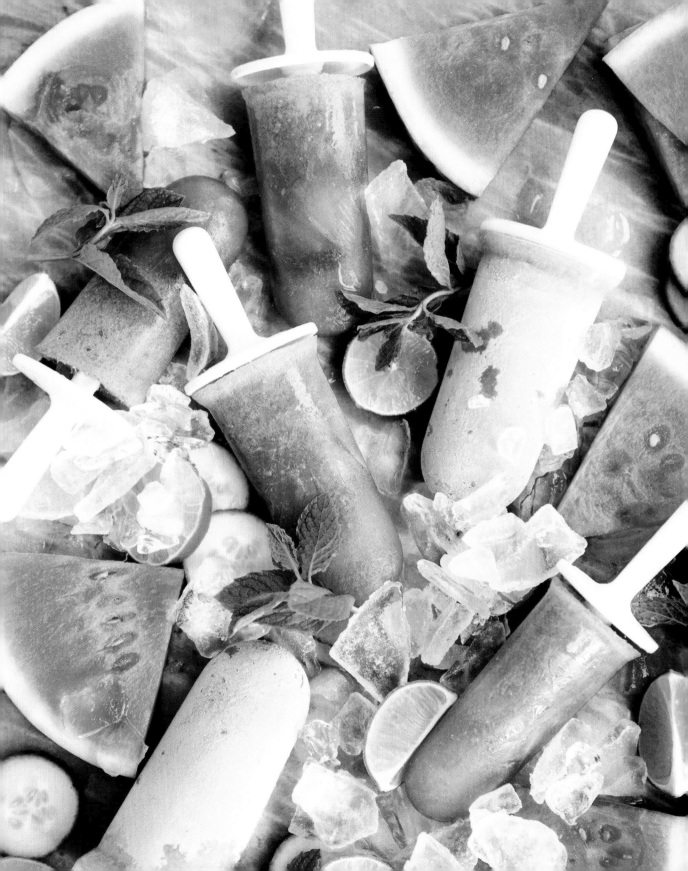

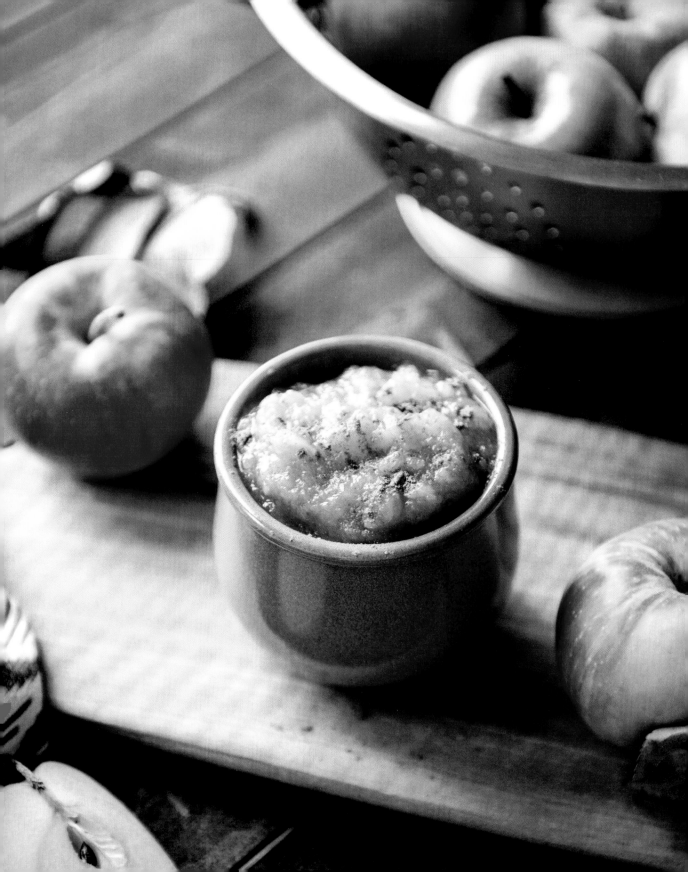

slow-cooker applesauce

When I started reading nutrition labels, I couldn't believe that 90 percent of the applesauce sold had corn syrup in it. I would be in the grocery store aisle talking out loud to myself about this. It blew my mind that a food so many kids were eating daily, and that was already naturally sweet, contained a hearty dose of corn syrup. Thankfully, there are a lot more options now, including unsweetened and organic, when it comes to applesauce products. Yet nothing compares to making it from scratch using fresh apples and a slow cooker. Throughout the day, the house begins to smell more and more delicious. **MAKES ABOUT 4½ CUPS**

5 pounds apples, peeled, cored, and roughly chopped

1 cup water

3 tablespoons fresh lemon juice (from 1 lemon)

2 cinnamon sticks

Pure maple syrup (optional)

1. In a slow cooker, combine the apples, water, lemon juice, and cinnamon sticks. Cook on low heat for 8 to 10 hours or on high for 4 to 5 hours, until the apples are cooked through.

2. Remove and discard the cinnamon sticks. Using an immersion blender, puree the applesauce to the desired consistency. Alternatively, mash the apples by hand.

3. Taste the applesauce. If it's not sweet enough, add maple syrup to taste.

GLUTEN FREE, NUT FREE, VEGAN, DAIRY FREE

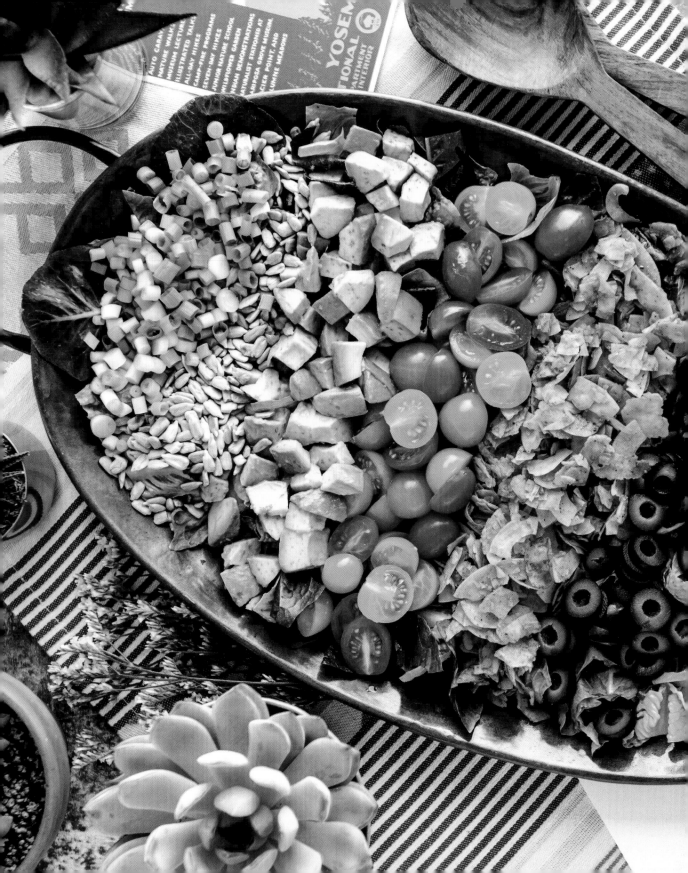

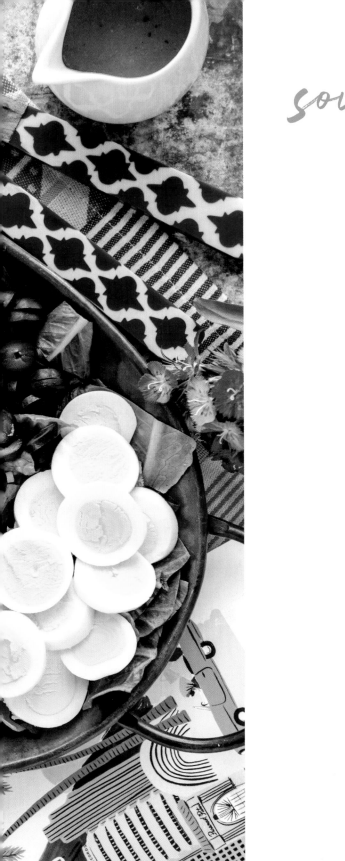

soups, salads, and sides

white bean soup

Most vegetarian soups don't keep me satisfied for very long, but this one is in a class of its own. Filled with plant-based protein, fiber, and carbs that nourish the soul and energize the body, this soup will keep you satisfied and full. Yet the best thing about this recipe is that it takes only one pot to make it. You can swap out the spinach for any of your favorite leafy greens. Kale and chard are both very good options; just make sure to remove the stems and roughly chop the leaves. **SERVES 6**

1 bag (16 ounces) dry cannellini beans, rinsed several times in cool water
2 carrots, peeled and diced
2 ribs celery, diced
1 yellow onion, diced
3 garlic cloves, minced
1 bay leaf
1 tablespoon Italian seasoning or Italian Herb Blend (page 194)

6 cups vegetable stock
1 cup water
1 can (28 ounces) organic diced tomatoes, undrained
Sea salt and ground black pepper
3 cups fresh spinach, roughly chopped
4 cups cooked brown rice, warmed

1. In a 4-quart or larger slow cooker, combine the beans, carrots, celery, onion, garlic, bay leaf, and Italian seasoning. Stir in the stock and water. Cover and cook on high for 3 hours or low for 6 hours.

2. Add the tomatoes and salt and pepper to taste. Cover and cook on high for 1½ hours or on low for 3 hours, or until the beans are tender.

3. Fifteen minutes before serving, stir in the spinach and let it wilt.

4. Ladle the soup into bowls along with a scoop of brown rice.

GLUTEN FREE, NUT FREE, VEGAN, DAIRY FREE

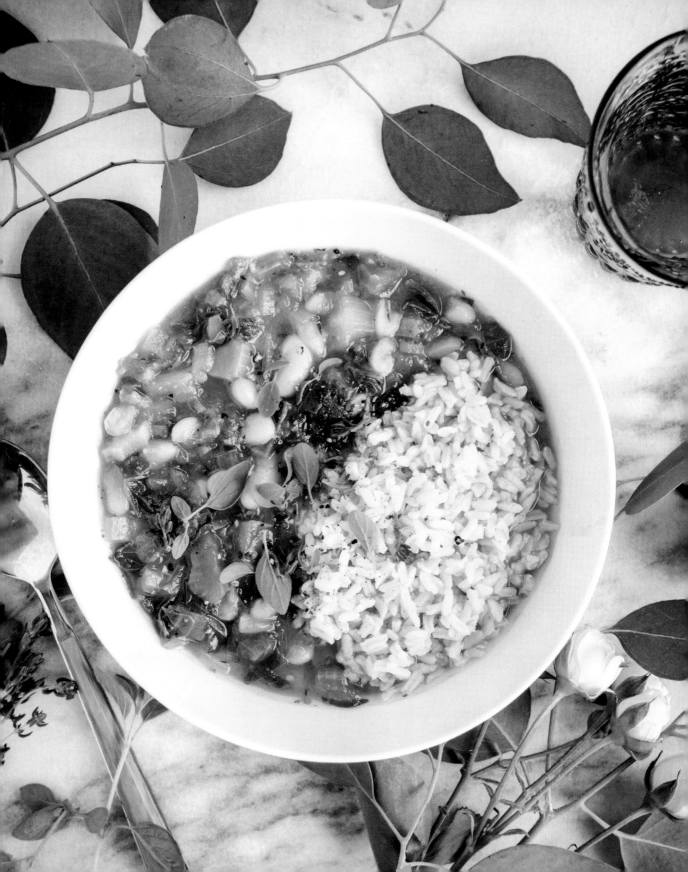

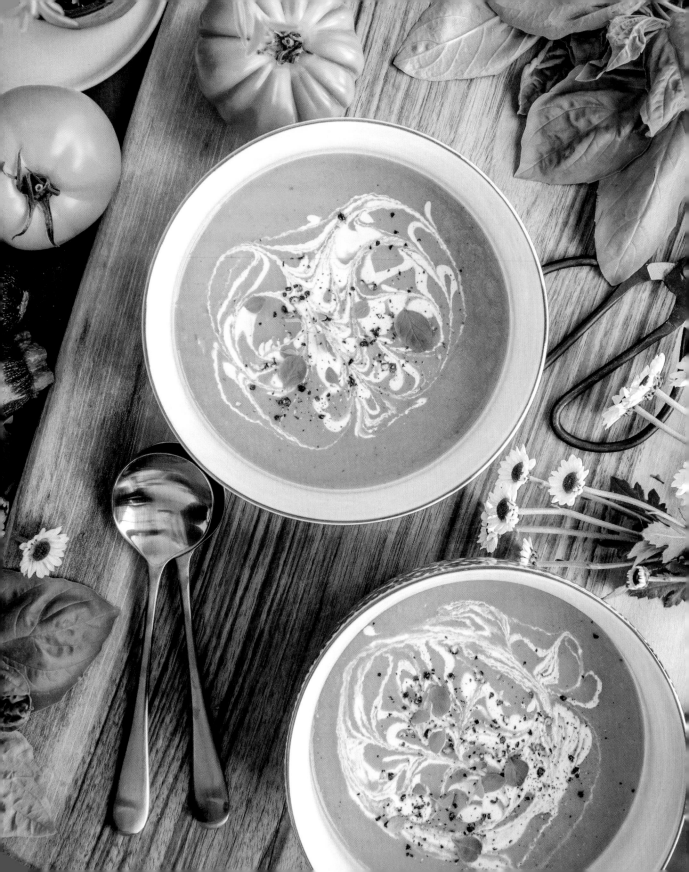

sneaky tomato soup

Late summer one year, Lindsey's garden was bountiful with zucchini and tomatoes. To use her produce before it went bad, she began sneaking zucchini into her tried-and-true tomato soup, and her kids didn't mind! Since then, I've brought this recipe into my home, and my family also approves. I've doctored it up with some of my favorite toppings. **SERVES 6**

1 tablespoon avocado oil
1 yellow onion, diced
Sea salt and ground black pepper
3 carrots, peeled and sliced
2 ribs celery, chopped
3 garlic cloves, minced
1 zucchini, sliced
4 cups vegetable stock

1 can (28 ounces) organic diced tomatoes, undrained
2 teaspoons Italian seasoning or Italian Herb Blend (page 194)

SUGGESTED TOPPINGS
Cashew Cream (page 67)
Fresh basil

1. In a 4-quart pot, warm the oil over medium-high heat. Add the onion and season with a little salt. Cook, stirring often, for 7 minutes, or until the onion starts to soften.

2. Add the carrots and celery and cook for 5 minutes, stirring occasionally. Then stir in the garlic and cook for 1 minute, or until fragrant. Add the zucchini and cook for a few minutes, until it starts to soften.

3. Stir in the stock, tomatoes, and Italian herbs. Bring just to a boil, then reduce the heat to low and simmer for 20 minutes, or until the vegetables are very soft and tender.

4. Using an immersion blender, or working carefully in batches with a standard blender, puree the soup. Season to taste with more salt and black pepper, if needed. Serve with your choice of toppings.

GLUTEN FREE, NUT FREE, VEGAN, DAIRY FREE

miso fine veggie bowl

I remember the first time I had miso soup—it was at my aunt and uncle's house in Redondo Beach. They had welcomed a Japanese woman, Akemi, into their home and she made us lunch one day—miso soup. My cousins quickly ate it like it was just another normal lunch, while I stared at it in confusion. What was this?! Yet after the first sip, I was hooked and slurped down the whole bowl. This recipe is a twist on that very soup and has gotten rave reviews from our rawkstar community. **SERVES 4**

¼ cup organic white miso paste
1 teaspoon sesame oil
6 cups vegetable stock, divided
1 tablespoon organic virgin coconut oil
1 cup thinly sliced scallions
1 tablespoon finely minced fresh ginger
3 garlic cloves, minced
1 cup thinly sliced shiitake mushrooms

½ cup shredded carrots
4 cups cored and very thinly sliced baby
   bok choy
1 zucchini, spiralized

FOR SERVING
4 hard-boiled eggs, halved
1 sheet nori, cut into thin strips (optional)

1. In a small bowl, stir together the miso and sesame oil. Add a little of the stock and stir to remove any lumps. Set aside.

2. In a large pot, warm the coconut oil over medium-high heat. Add the scallions and cook, stirring constantly, for 2 minutes, or until bright green. Add the ginger and garlic and cook, stirring constantly, for 30 to 60 seconds.

3. Add the mushrooms and carrots. Keep cooking, stirring occasionally, for 3 minutes, then add the bok choy and sauté briefly.

4. Stir in the miso mixture and the remaining stock. Bring to a simmer and cook for a few minutes so the flavors blend. Add the zucchini noodles and allow them to soften in the broth.

5. To serve, ladle the soup into bowls and top each with 2 hard-boiled egg halves and a sprinkling of nori strips, if using. Serve immediately.

GLUTEN FREE, NUT FREE, VEGAN *(remove the eggs)*, DAIRY FREE

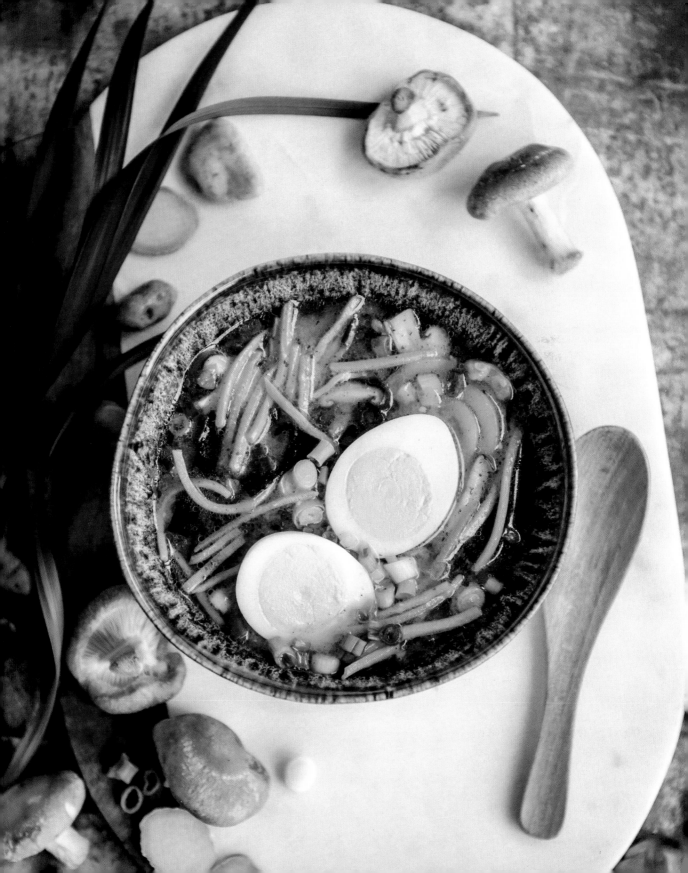

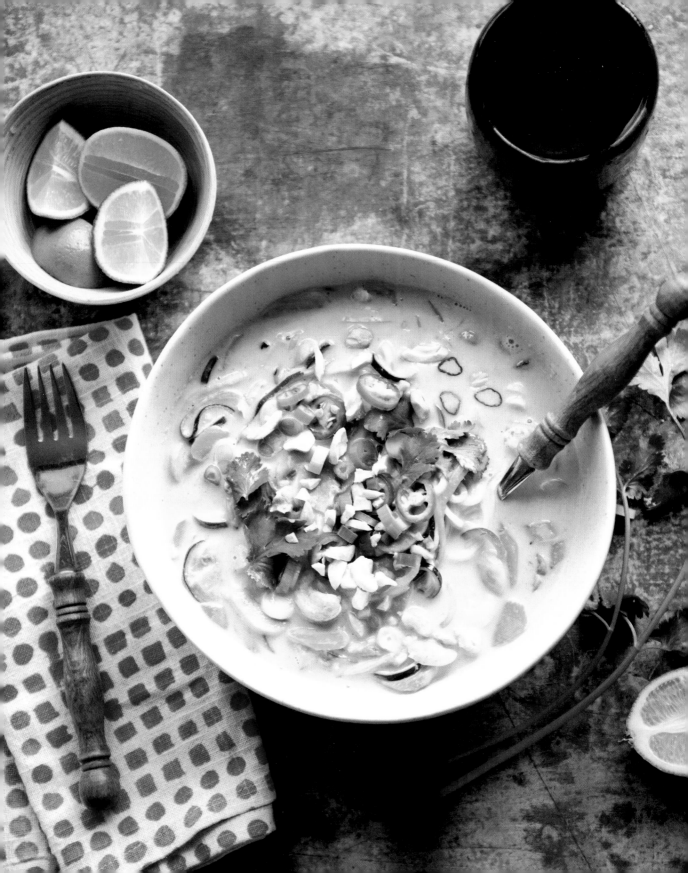

coconut thai soup

This recipe is from our Thrive: A 7-Day Reset program (http://sgs.to/thrive). It's my favorite soup of all time—and many rawkstars will agree! I had no clue how deep my love for soup could go until I made this one. I've brought it to dinner parties, and it's always a hit. **SERVES 4**

4 cans (13 ounces each) full-fat
   coconut milk
4 tablespoons red or green Thai
   curry paste
2 teaspoons pure maple syrup
½ teaspoon sea salt
1 cup very thinly sliced carrots
1 cup thinly sliced baby bella
   mushrooms
2 zucchini, spiralized

FOR SERVING
½ cup raw cashews, chopped
¼ cup sliced scallions
1 serrano chile pepper, thinly sliced
1 lime, cut into wedges

1. In a large saucepan, whisk together the coconut milk and curry paste. Bring to a simmer over medium heat. Stir in the maple syrup and salt. Add the carrots and mushrooms and simmer for 20 minutes, or until the carrots are tender. Add the zucchini noodles. Taste and add more salt, if needed.

2. Ladle into serving bowls and garnish with cashews, scallions, chile pepper, and lime wedges. Serve immediately.

GLUTEN FREE, NUT FREE *(remove the cashews)*, VEGAN, DAIRY FREE

fiesta soup

Sautéed onions and bell peppers bring out the deep flavors in this Mexican soup. I could eat this every single day for lunch and never get sick of it! Definitely add the avocado, lime, and cilantro to brighten the flavors and provide a creamy texture and spicy bite.   **SERVES 6**

1 tablespoon avocado oil
1 yellow onion, diced
1 red bell pepper, diced
1 zucchini, diced
3 garlic cloves, minced
2 tablespoons taco seasoning or
    Simple Taco Seasoning (page 107)
4 cups vegetable stock
1 can (15 ounces) black beans, drained
    and rinsed
1 can (15 ounces) pinto beans, drained
    and rinsed

1 can (15 ounces) organic diced
    tomatoes, undrained
1 can (7 ounces) diced green chiles
1 cup organic frozen corn
2 tablespoons fresh lime juice
    (from 1 lime)
¼ cup fresh cilantro, chopped
Sea salt and ground black pepper

FOR SERVING
½ cup organic corn tortilla strips
3 ripe avocados, diced
½ cup fresh cilantro, roughly chopped
1 lime, cut into wedges

1. Heat a large pot over medium-high heat. Add the oil and let it warm for 30 seconds, then add the onion and bell pepper. Cook, stirring frequently, for 5 minutes, or until the bell peppers start to brown and the onions turn translucent. Add the zucchini and garlic and cook for 1 minute, until fragrant. Add the taco seasoning and cook, stirring constantly, for a bit longer to toast the spices.

2. Add the stock, beans, tomatoes, and chiles. Stir well. Bring just to a boil, then reduce the heat to low and simmer for 20 minutes, or until the flavors blend and veggies become tender.

3. Stir in the corn, lime juice, and cilantro and season with salt and black pepper. Remove from the heat. Ladle into bowls, top with some of the tortilla strips, avocado, and cilantro, and serve with a lime wedge.

GLUTEN FREE, NUT FREE, VEGAN, DAIRY FREE

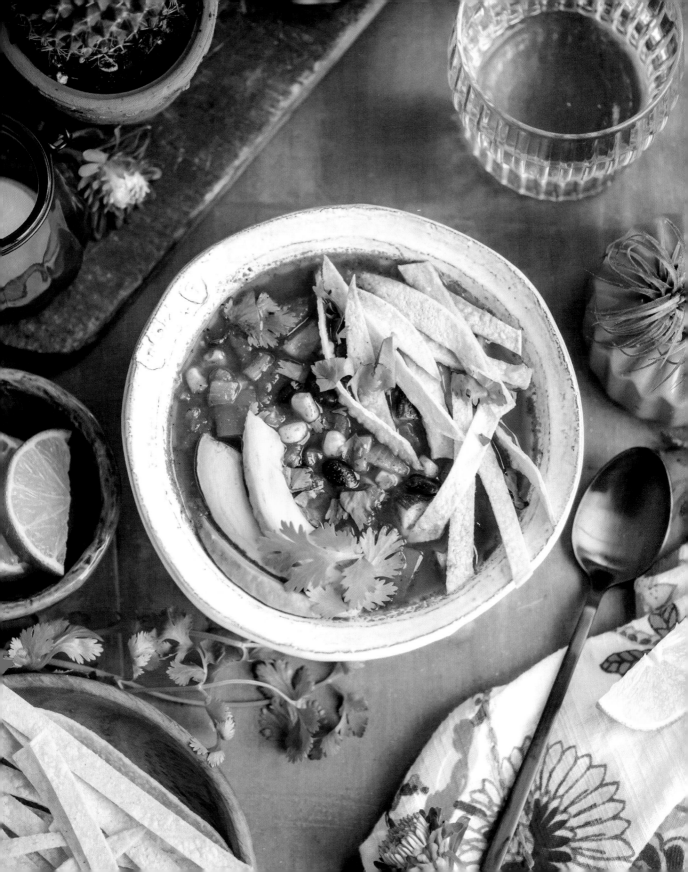

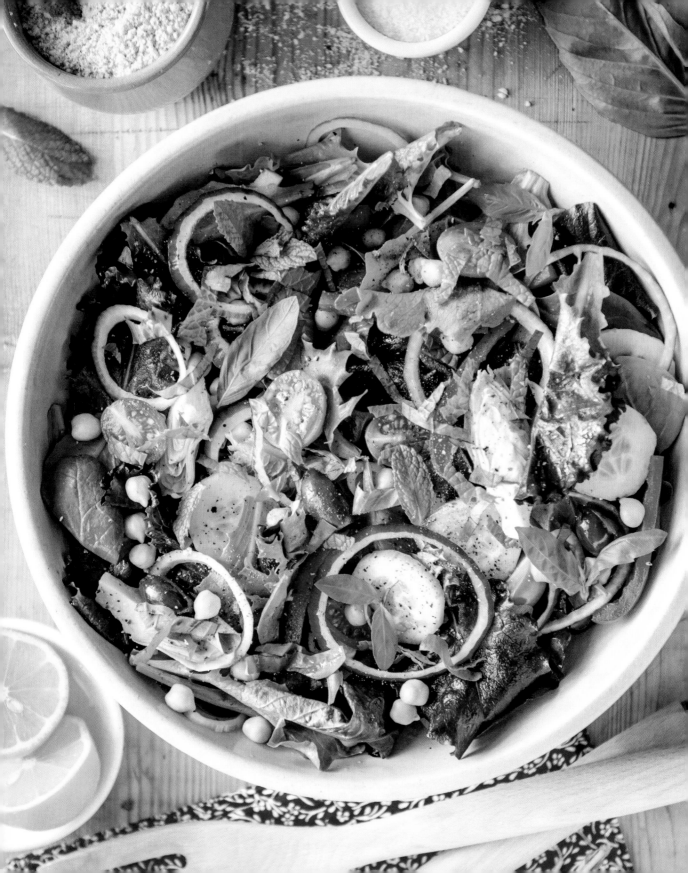

the hungry greek salad

I love a good salad, but what I love even more are the toppings that go on a good salad. This one is a favorite with a ton of tasty herbs, spices, and marinated veggies that take a good salad and make it great. **SERVES 4**

8 cups mixed greens
1 cup canned chickpeas, drained and rinsed
½ cucumber, sliced
1 red bell pepper, sliced
1 cup grape tomatoes, halved
½ cup marinated artichoke hearts, drained and chopped
½ cup thinly sliced red onion

½ cup kalamata olives, pitted
3 tablespoons extra-virgin olive oil
3 tablespoons fresh lemon juice (from 1 lemon)
Sea salt and ground black pepper
¼ cup chopped fresh basil, oregano, and mint
¼ cup Cheeze Sprinkle (page 151)

1. In a large serving bowl, make a base with the greens. Layer the chickpeas, cucumber, bell pepper, tomatoes, artichoke hearts, onion, and olives on top of the greens.

2. Drizzle the oil and lemon juice over the salad, season with salt and black pepper, and sprinkle on the fresh herbs. Gently toss.

3. Serve the cheeze sprinkle on the side.

GLUTEN FREE, NUT FREE, VEGAN, DAIRY FREE

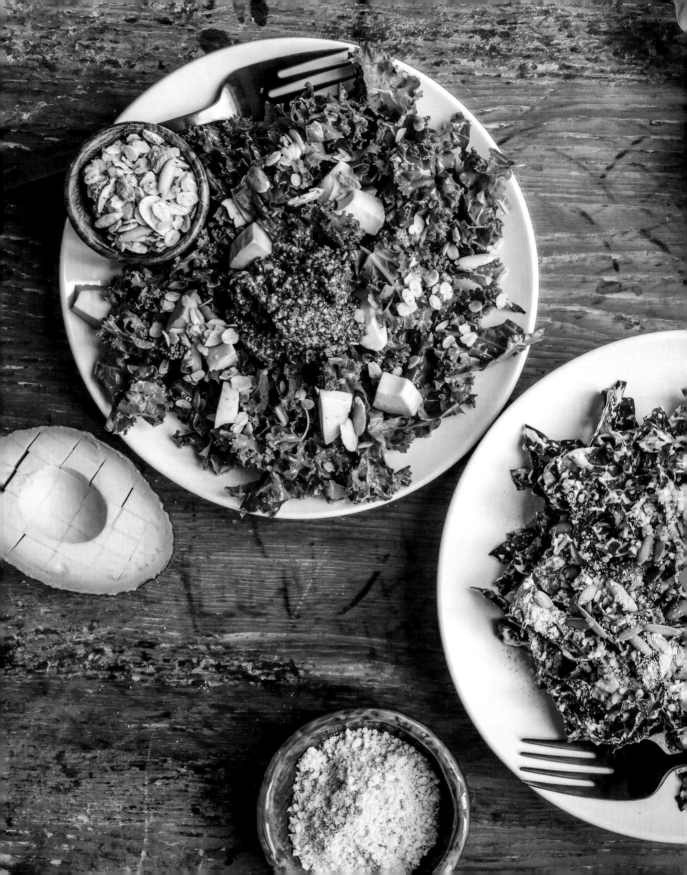

kale yeah

I thought kale chips were the most amazing thing
that could be done with that particular bitter leafy
green until I tried a massaged kale salad. Holy
kale—it's amazing! The trick is to massage those
kale leaves to get them nice and tender. Then
smother them with a tasty dressing and topping
and you have a filling, fiber-rich meal.

Now, when you first read that instruction to
massage your salad, you may have heard your
mother's voice whisper in your ear, "Don't play with
your food." But massaging kale actually softens
the texture so that the leaves are more enjoyable
to eat! The process subdues kale's bitter taste—
something that otherwise requires long, slow
cooking to reduce.

raw-ish kale caesar salad SERVES 4

1 bunch kale, stems removed and thinly
  sliced into ribbons
2 tablespoons extra-virgin olive oil
3 tablespoons fresh lemon juice
  (from 1 lemon)
Sea salt and ground black pepper

1 can (15 ounces) chickpeas, drained and
  rinsed
½ cup Cashew-Garlic Aioli (below)
¼ cup pepitas
¼ cup Cheeze Sprinkle (page 151)

1. Place the kale in a large serving bowl and drizzle it with the oil. With clean hands,
   gently massage the kale and oil for 5 minutes, or until the kale is tenderized. Squeeze
   the lemon juice over the top and season well with salt and black pepper to taste.

2. Add the chickpeas and aioli and toss until well combined.

3. Divide between 4 plates and sprinkle each with pepitas and cheeze sprinkle. Serve
   immediately.

CASHEW-GARLIC AIOLI MAKES ABOUT 1 CUP

1 cup raw cashews
5 tablespoons fresh lemon juice, divided
3 garlic cloves

1 teaspoon Dijon mustard
¼ teaspoon sea salt, or more to taste

1. Place the cashews in a medium bowl and pour 2 tablespoons of the lemon juice over the
   top. Add enough water to cover by a few inches. Let soak for 2 hours, then drain and rinse
   well.

2. In a blender, combine the cashews, garlic, mustard, salt, and the remaining 3 tablespoons
   lemon juice. Pulse a few times, then blend on low. If needed, add a few tablespoons water.
   The mixture should be thick and creamy, sorta like mayonnaise (as much as I struggle with
   that visual). Taste and add more salt or lemon juice as desired.

3. Transfer to an airtight container and refrigerate. This keeps well up to 1 week in the fridge
   or up to several months in the freezer.

GLUTEN FREE, NUT FREE *(omit the aioli)*, VEGAN, DAIRY FREE

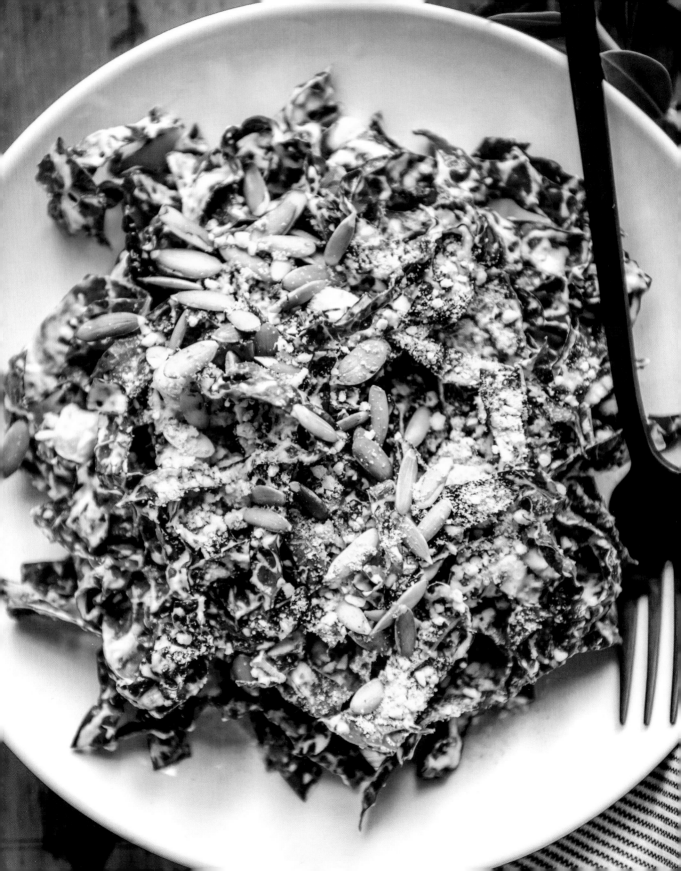

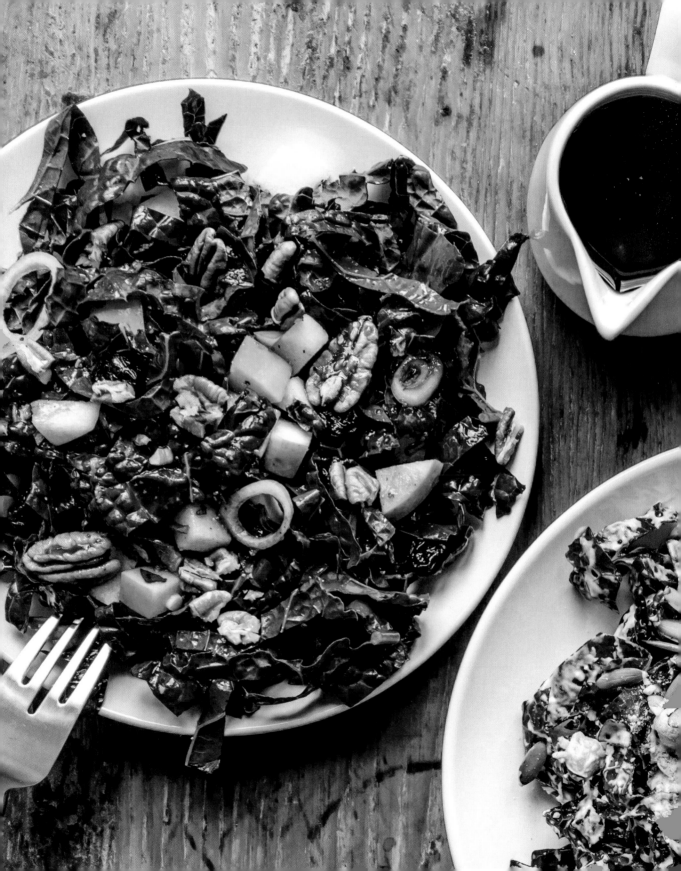

fruit 'n' nut kale salad SERVES 4

1 bunch kale, stems removed and thinly
    sliced into ribbons
2 tablespoons extra-virgin olive oil
3 tablespoons fresh lemon juice
    (from 1 lemon)
Sea salt and ground black pepper

1 green apple, cored and diced
½ cup dried tart cherries
½ cup pecans, chopped
1 shallot, very thinly sliced into rings
½ cup Balsamic Herb Vinaigrette
    (below)

1. Place the kale in a large serving bowl and drizzle it with the oil. With clean hands, gently massage the kale and oil for 5 minutes, or until the kale is tenderized. Pour the lemon juice over the top and season well with salt and pepper to taste.

2. Add the apple, cherries, pecans, and shallot, drizzle in a little of the dressing, and toss well.

3. Divide between 4 plates and serve immediately.

BALSAMIC HERB VINAIGRETTE MAKES ABOUT 1 CUP

⅓ cup balsamic vinegar
1 tablespoon chopped fresh thyme
1 tablespoon chopped fresh rosemary
1 tablespoon chopped fresh sage
1 teaspoon honey

½ teaspoon Dijon mustard
½ teaspoon sea salt
¼ teaspoon ground black pepper
Pinch of garlic powder
⅔ cup extra-virgin olive oil

1. In a pint mason jar, combine the vinegar, thyme, rosemary, sage, honey, mustard, salt, pepper, and garlic powder. Attach the lid and shake until well combined.

2. Add the oil to the jar, reattach the lid, and shake again. Store in the fridge for 1 to 2 weeks.

GLUTEN FREE, NUT FREE *(remove the pecans)*, VEGAN *(replace honey in dressing with maple syrup)*, DAIRY FREE

pesto–raw kale salad SERVES 4

1 bunch kale, stems removed and thinly
  sliced into ribbons
2 tablespoons extra-virgin olive oil
3 tablespoons fresh lemon juice
Sea salt and ground black pepper

FOR TOPPING
4 tablespoons Basil Pesto (page 139)
1 ripe avocado, diced
½ cup Savory Granola (below)

1. Place the kale in a large serving bowl and drizzle it with the oil. With clean hands, gently massage the kale and oil for 5 minutes, or until the kale is tenderized. Pour the lemon juice over the top and season well with salt and pepper to taste.

2. Divide the kale among 4 plates. Top each with a heaping tablespoon of pesto, some diced avocado, and 2 tablespoons granola. Serve immediately.

GLUTEN FREE, NUT FREE *(top with avocado only and leave nuts out of pesto)*, VEGAN, DAIRY FREE

savory granola SERVES 8

3 cups gluten-free rolled oats
½ cup sliced raw almonds
½ cup raw sunflower seeds
½ cup raw pepitas
¼ cup almond meal
6 tablespoons avocado oil
2 tablespoons pure maple syrup

2 teaspoons dried rosemary
1 teaspoon dried thyme
½ teaspoon dry mustard powder
½ teaspoon sea salt
½ teaspoon onion powder
¼ teaspoon garlic powder
¼ teaspoon ground black pepper

1. Preheat the oven to 350°F.

2. In a large bowl, combine all the ingredients and stir well. Spread evenly on a rimmed baking sheet. Bake for 15 to 20 minutes, or until toasted. Remove and let cool completely, then transfer to an airtight container.

GLUTEN FREE, NUT FREE *(replace ¼ cup almond meal with ¼ cup ground flaxseed or flax meal)*, VEGAN, DAIRY FREE

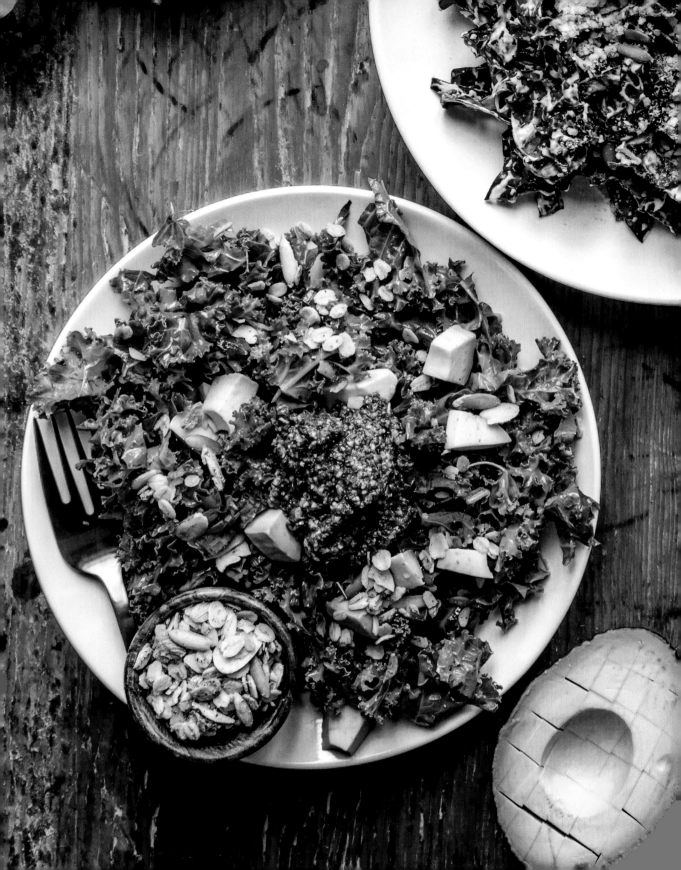

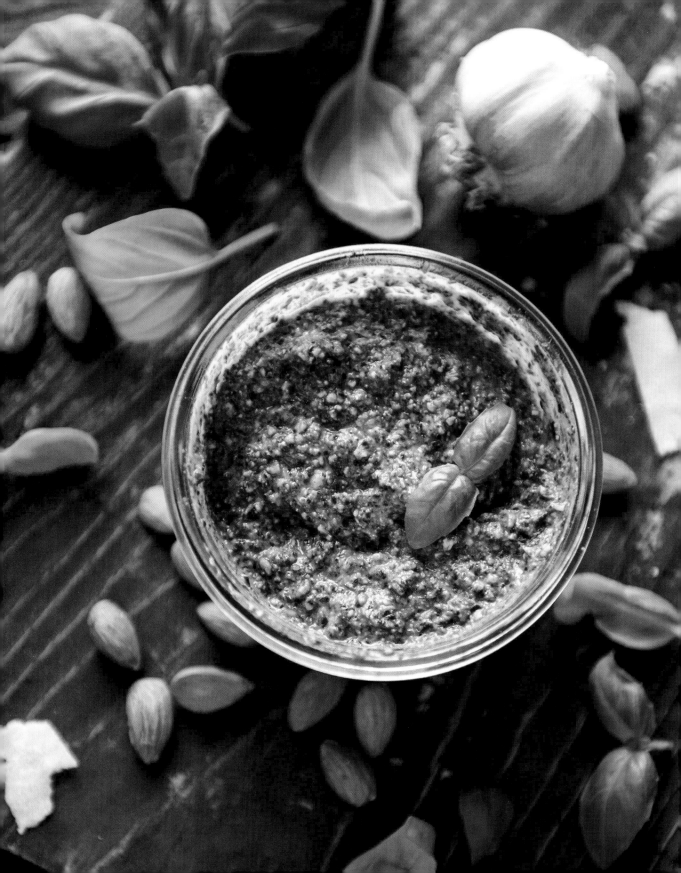

basil pesto SERVES 4

½ cup pine nuts
3 garlic cloves, halved
6 cups fresh basil leaves, gently packed
   (about 2 large bunches)

¼ teaspoon sea salt
½ cup extra-virgin olive oil

1. In a food processor fitted with the chopping blade, combine the pine nuts and garlic and pulse until finely chopped. Add the basil and salt and pulse again until finely chopped.

2. With the motor running, pour the oil through the feed hole in a slow, steady stream. Process until smooth. Stop to scrape down the sides, if needed, while processing.

3. Transfer to an airtight container and refrigerate until ready to use. It will keep about 1 week in the fridge or up to several months in the freezer.

GLUTEN FREE, VEGAN, DAIRY FREE

summer quinoa salad

My friends Susan and Ginna brought their mom to a church potluck, and she contributed a kale-quinoa salad that rawked my world. I ended up eating 90 percent of it—it was *sooooo* good! I asked what was in it and now make my own. This is a great side dish for any potluck or barbecue or just a light lunch during the week. **SERVES 4**

1 cup dry quinoa
2 cups vegetable stock
2 tablespoons balsamic vinegar
1 tablespoon extra-virgin olive oil
1 tablespoon fresh lemon juice
Sea salt and ground black pepper

¼ cup raisins, soaked in water for 10 minutes and drained
1 carrot, finely grated
1 cup kale, stems removed and thinly sliced
2 scallions, thickly sliced
2 tablespoons sunflower seeds
2 tablespoons pepitas

1. If the quinoa is not prerinsed (check the package), place it in a fine-mesh sieve and rinse well with cool water to remove the bitter saponins on the quinoa. Drain well.

2. In a medium pot, combine the quinoa and stock. Bring to a boil, then reduce the heat to low and cover the pot. Cook for 20 minutes, or until the quinoa is cooked through. Let stand for 10 minutes, then transfer the quinoa to a shallow freezer container and place in the freezer for 20 minutes to quickly cool it.

3. Meanwhile, in a small bowl, make the dressing by whisking together the vinegar, oil, and lemon juice and season with salt and pepper to taste.

4. When the quinoa is chilled, transfer it to a medium bowl. Add the raisins, carrot, kale, scallions, sunflower seeds, and pepitas. Drizzle the dressing on top of the salad and toss well to combine.

GLUTEN FREE, NUT FREE, VEGAN, DAIRY FREE

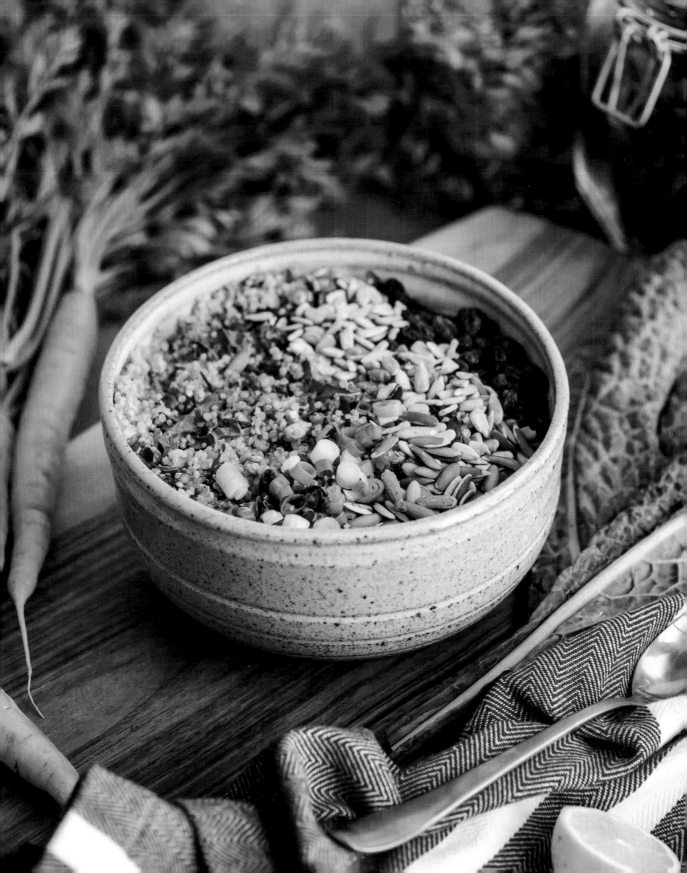

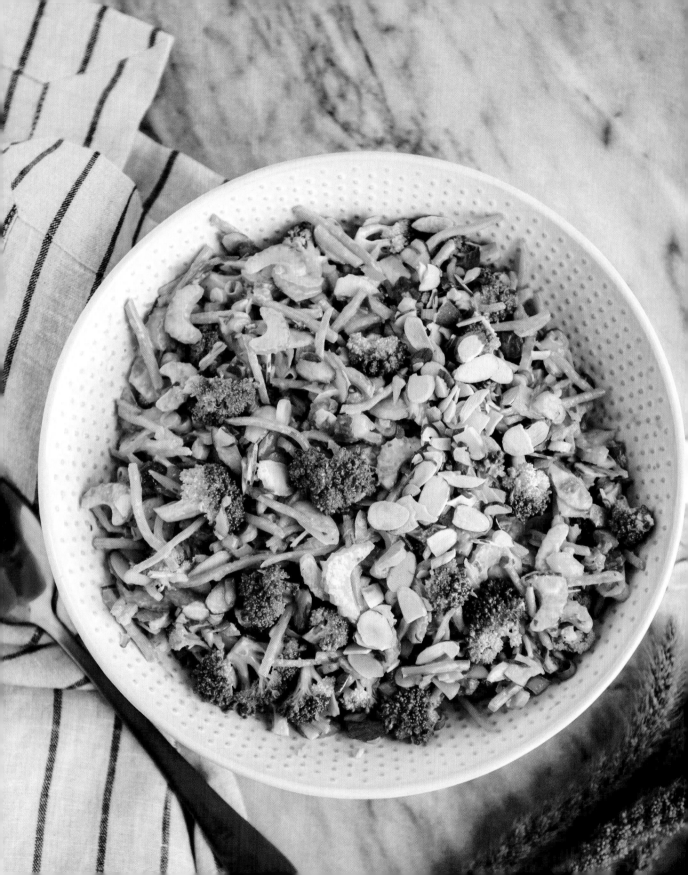

tiny trees salad

When my kids were teeny tiny, I used to pretend that broccoli was a forest of trees and we'd admire them before each bite. That's how I got my kids to love broccoli and happily eat it to this day. This salad takes raw broccoli to a whole new level, coated in a rich savory sauce and combined with celery and carrots. It's intended as a side dish, but I have been known to eat it for lunch. **SERVES 4**

1 head broccoli, chopped into florets
1 cup thinly sliced scallions
1 cup thinly sliced celery

1 cup shredded carrots
1 cup sliced almonds
Sweet Tahini Dressing (below)

In a salad bowl, combine the broccoli, scallions, celery, carrots, and almonds. Pour the dressing on top and toss until well coated. Cover and refrigerate until ready to serve.

SWEET TAHINI DRESSING MAKES ¾ CUP

¼ cup tahini
¼ cup fresh orange juice
2 tablespoons tamari

1 tablespoon pure maple syrup
2 teaspoons sesame oil
2 garlic cloves, finely minced

In a medium bowl, whisk together the tahini, orange juice, tamari, maple syrup, oil, and minced garlic. Store in an airtight container until ready to use.

GLUTEN FREE, NUT FREE *(replace sliced almonds with pepitas)*, VEGAN, DAIRY FREE

grilled veggie kabobs

On a hot summer day in Florida, the last thing I want to do is turn on the oven and heat up the house. The grill becomes our summer kitchen and where a lot of veggie action happens. These veggies kabobs are simple staples, but they become out of this world when drizzled with the yummy sauces. **SERVES 4**

1 zucchini, cut into ½-inch-thick rounds

½ cup baby bella or white button mushrooms, stems removed

1 red or yellow bell pepper, cut into 1-inch chunks

½ red onion, cut into 1-inch chunks

2 cups cherry tomatoes

2 tablespoons avocado oil

Sea salt and ground black pepper

FOR SERVING

Almond Butter Sauce (page 198)

Coconut Sriracha Sauce (page 61)

Cashew Ranch Dipping Sauce (page 168)

1. If using bamboo skewers, soak the skewers in water for 30 minutes. (Skip this step if using metal skewers.)

2. Preheat a grill to medium-high or heat a grill pan on the stove.

3. Thread the zucchini, mushrooms, bell pepper, onion, and tomatoes onto the skewers. Drizzle a little of the oil over the kebabs and season well with salt and black pepper to taste.

4. Grill the kabobs for 7 minutes, then turn them and grill for 5 to 7 minutes, or until the veggies are tender-crisp.

5. Remove from the grill, season again with a little salt and black pepper, and serve warm with sauces on the side.

GLUTEN FREE, NUT FREE *(do not use nut sauces)*, VEGAN, DAIRY FREE

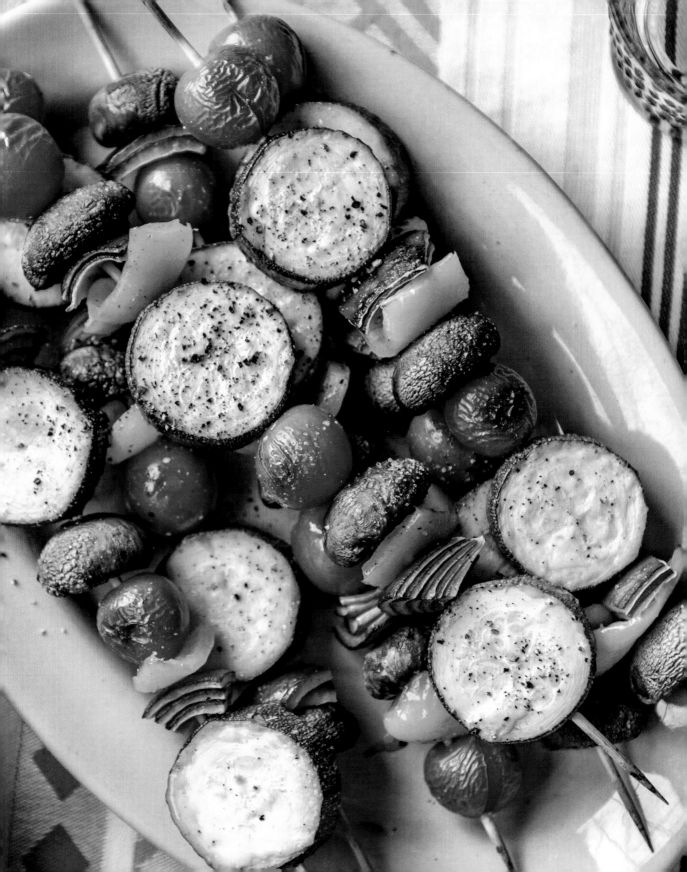

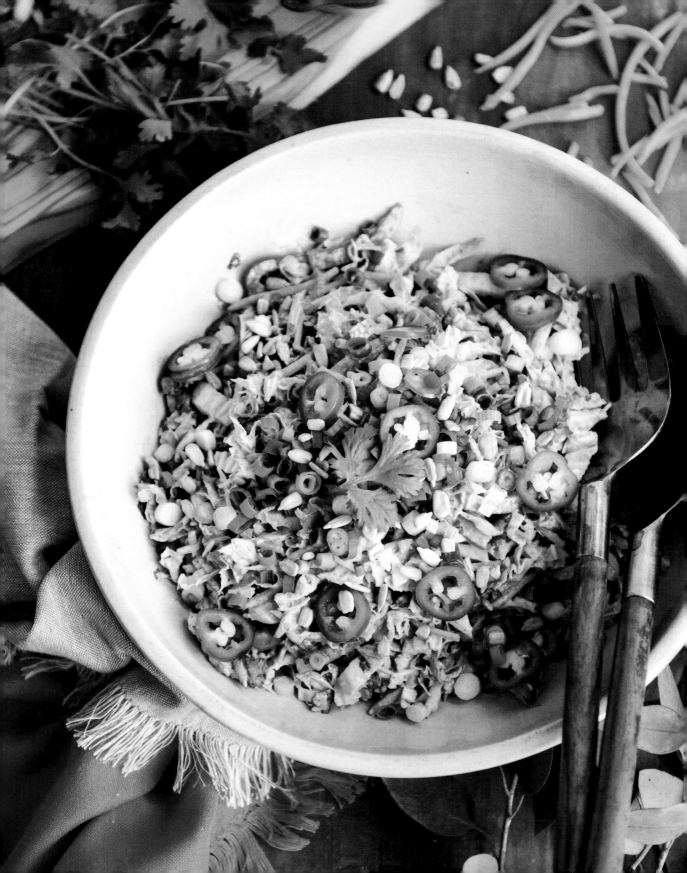

crunchy curry salad

Last year, I started getting into endurance running and immersed myself in Scott Jurek's book, *Eat and Run*. He's an amazing vegan ultra-distance runner, and he shared some great recipes throughout his story. This Crunchy Curry Cabbage Slaw is adapted from a recipe in his book that really stood out and has become a favorite of mine. **SERVES 4**

1 head napa cabbage	¼ cup canned full-fat coconut milk
1 cup shredded carrots	¼ cup rice vinegar
1 red bell pepper, julienned	¼ cup diced yellow onion
½ cup thinly sliced scallions	2 tablespoons white miso paste
½ cup fresh cilantro, roughly chopped	2 tablespoons pure maple syrup
½ cup sunflower seeds	1 tablespoon red curry paste
1 jalapeño chile pepper, thickly sliced	1 garlic clove, minced
½ cup creamy almond butter	½-inch piece fresh ginger, peeled

1. Trim the end of the cabbage, halve and core it, and cut into very thin ribbons, or shred. Place in a bowl with the carrots, bell pepper, scallions, cilantro, sunflower seeds, and chile pepper. Set aside.

2. In a blender, make a curry sauce by combining the almond butter, coconut milk, vinegar, onion, miso, maple syrup, curry paste, garlic, and ginger and puree until smooth. Stop to scrape down the sides as needed. If the mixture is too thick, add a little more coconut milk and blend again.

3. Pour the sauce over the cabbage mixture. Toss well to combine. Serve immediately or store in an airtight container for up to 5 days.

GLUTEN FREE, NUT FREE, VEGAN, DAIRY FREE

simple cashew coleslaw

I've always been a coleslaw lover but struggled these last few years as I've moved away from mayonnaise and most processed foods. This plant-based rendition has an amazing crunch and a sweet and creamy bite that tastes even better than traditional coleslaw to me, and it's perfect for the Austinite Tacos (page 197). **SERVES 4**

½ head napa cabbage, cored and
  shredded
¼ cup shredded carrots
½ cup Cashew-Garlic Aioli
  (page 132)

1 tablespoon apple cider vinegar, or
  more to taste
2 teaspoons coconut sugar
¼ teaspoon sea salt

In a mixing bowl, combine the cabbage and carrots. Add the aioli, vinegar, coconut sugar, and salt. Toss until well combined, then refrigerate until ready to serve.

GLUTEN FREE, NUT FREE *(replace the aioli with ½ cup vegan mayo)*, VEGAN, DAIRY FREE

rawkstar tip

Distilled white vinegar or lemon juice can be used in place of the apple cider vinegar. You can also swap out the coconut sugar for maple syrup or honey.

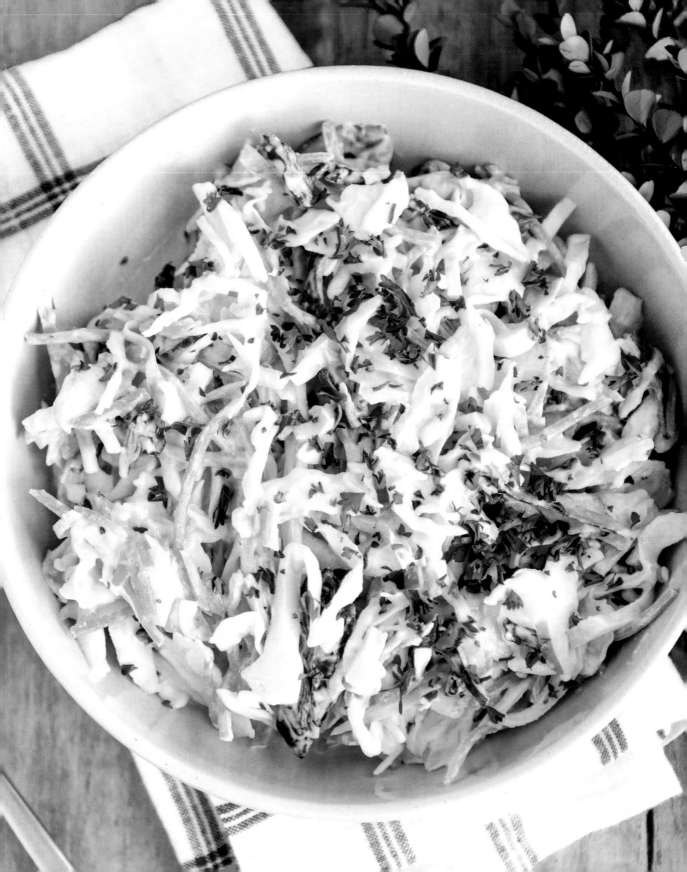

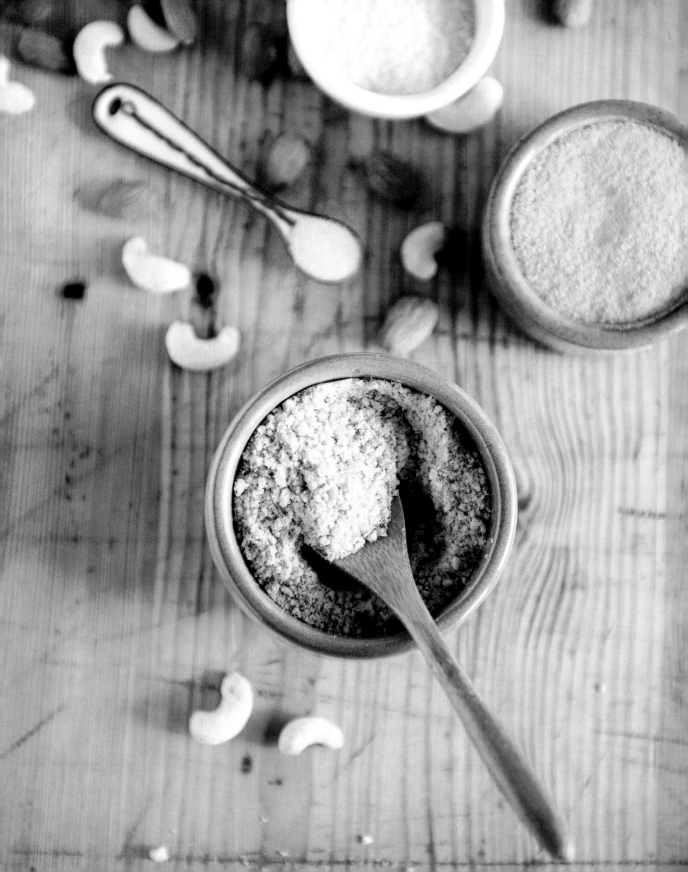

cheeze sprinkle

I love cheese, but it doesn't always love me. It slows down my digestive system and causes my tummy to talk loudly as Ryan and I are lying in bed at night. Occasionally, it's worth the side effects to enjoy some good cheese . . . and other times it's not. This cheese substitute is easy enough to whip up and keep on hand for the days when I need a cheese alternative for a burrito, soup, or salad, or on top of my popcorn during our family Friday movie night. **MAKES ABOUT ¾ CUP**

½ cup raw almonds
½ cup raw cashews
¼ cup nutritional yeast

½ teaspoon sea salt
¼ teaspoon garlic powder

1. In a food processor, combine the nuts, nutritional yeast, salt, and garlic powder and pulse until finely chopped. The mixture should look like bread crumbs.

2. Transfer to an airtight container and store in a cool, dry place or the refrigerator for up to several weeks.

GLUTEN FREE, VEGAN, DAIRY FREE

california cobb salad

When life gives you romaine lettuce, you make a plant-powered cobb salad. I take this salad very seriously and made sure to include some coconut bacon and creamy dressing to delight the tastebuds and leave you California dreamin'. **SERVES 4**

1 head romaine lettuce, chopped
1 cup cherry tomatoes, halved
½ cup black olives, sliced
4 hard-boiled eggs, sliced
2 ripe avocados, diced

¾ cup Coconut Bacon (page 80)
½ cup thinly sliced scallions
½ cup toasted sunflower seeds
2 tablespoons Creamy Herb Dressing (below)

Place the lettuce on a large serving platter or in a wide, shallow salad bowl. Arrange the tomatoes, olives, eggs, avocados, bacon, scallions, and sunflower seeds in horizontal rows over the lettuce. Drizzle the salad with the vinaigrette or dressing. Serve immediately.

CREAMY HERB DRESSING

MAKES ¾ CUP

1 yellow onion, diced
2 tablespoons fresh lemon juice
1 teaspoon pure maple syrup
1 teaspoon Dijon mustard
1 garlic clove

½ teaspoon sea salt
½ teaspoon ground black pepper
½ cup extra-virgin olive oil
¼ cup finely chopped fresh dill
¼ cup finely chopped fresh parsley

1. In a blender, combine the onion, lemon juice, maple syrup, mustard, garlic, salt, and pepper and puree until smooth, stopping to scrape down the sides as needed.

2. With the motor running, pour the oil through the feed hole and blend until smooth and creamy. Pour into a widemouthed jar and add the dill and parsley. Shake well.

3. Store in the refrigerator for up to 1 week.

GLUTEN FREE, NUT FREE, VEGAN *(remove the eggs)*, DAIRY FREE

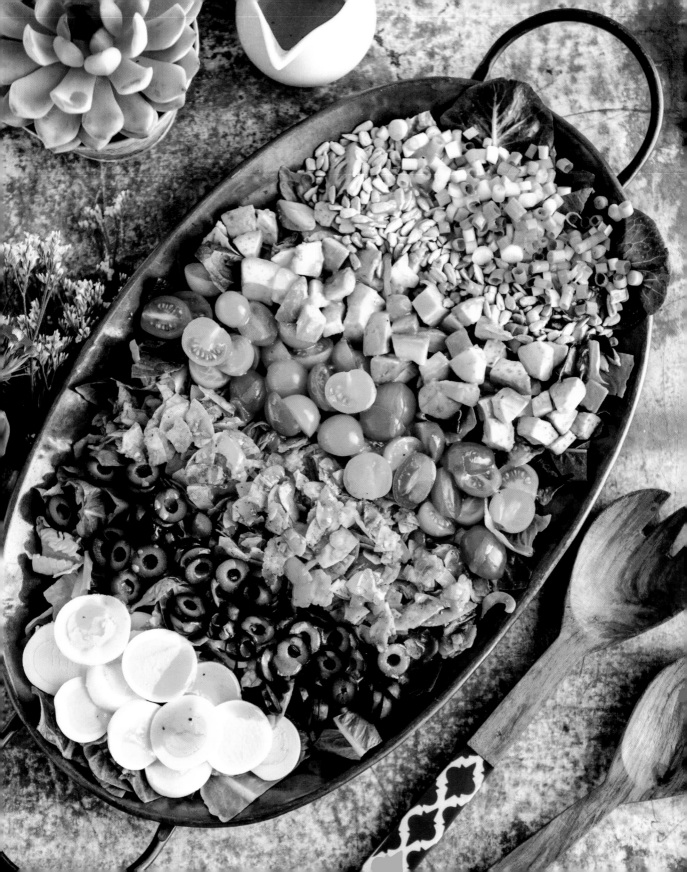

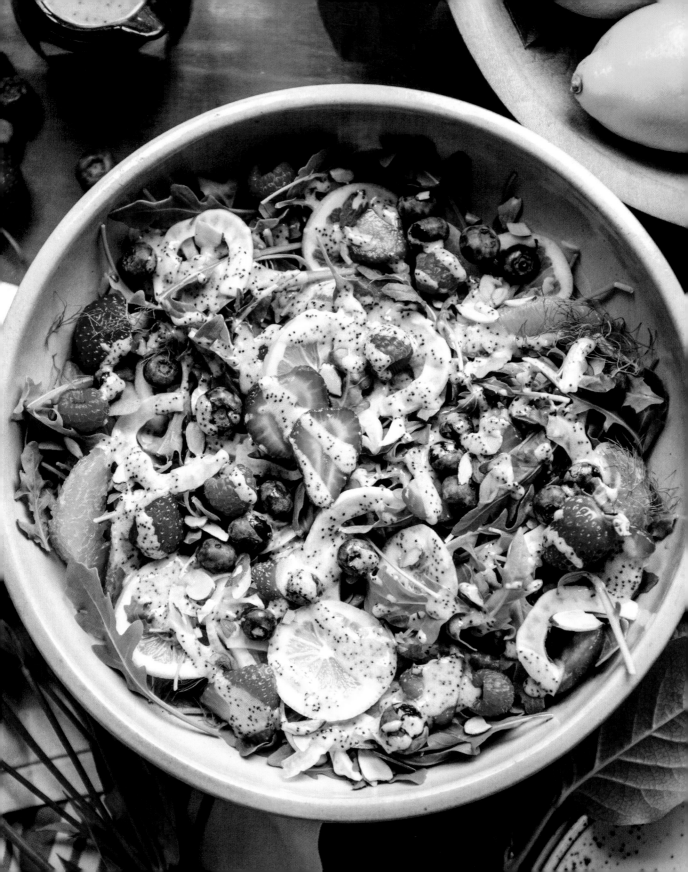

berry sunshine salad

This salad is pretty much sunshine over a field of greens on a plate to alkalize your body. The triple-berry medley adds a boost of antioxidants, color, and sweetness to keep any sugar cravings at bay, while the lemon and fennel come together to create a light, refreshing palate cleanser. Each bite is better than the last! **SERVES 4**

8 cups baby arugula
1 medium fennel bulb, very thinly sliced
2 oranges, peeled and segmented
1 cup strawberries, sliced
1 cup blueberries

1 cup raspberries
1 Meyer lemon, seeded and very thinly sliced
½ cup sliced almonds
Meyer Lemon Dressing (below)

In a large salad bowl, combine the arugula, fennel, oranges, berries, lemon, and almonds. Drizzle a little of the dressing over the salad and toss to coat. Divide between 4 plates and serve with the remaining dressing on the side.

MEYER LEMON DRESSING

MAKES ABOUT ¾ CUP

¼ cup Cashew Cream (page 67)
¼ cup fresh Meyer lemon juice
1 tablespoon honey
½ teaspoon sea salt

Big pinch of ground black pepper
¼ cup extra-virgin olive oil
1 tablespoon poppy seeds

1. In a blender, combine the cashew cream, lemon juice, honey, salt, and pepper and puree until smooth, stopping to scrape down the sides as needed.

2. With the motor running, pour the oil through the feed hole and blend until smooth and creamy. Pour into a jar with a tight-fitting lid and stir in the poppy seeds. Attach the lid and store in the refrigerator for up to 1 week.

GLUTEN FREE, NUT FREE *(replace almonds with sunflower seeds)*, VEGAN *(replace honey in dressing with pure maple syrup)*, DAIRY FREE

autumn salad in a jar

I'm never that excited to eat salads as it turns to fall and then winter. But I know the health benefits are for real, so I've learned a few tricks to keep me going with the greens: I add seasonal ingredients that give my salads substance and depth. The chickpeas, butternut squash, and pomegranate in this recipe are a true celebration of autumn. **SERVES 2**

1 cup cubed butternut squash
(½-inch cubes)
2 tablespoons organic virgin coconut oil, melted
½ cup dry quinoa
1 cup vegetable stock

1 cup canned chickpeas, rinsed and drained
2 cups kale, stems removed and thinly sliced
4 tablespoons pomegranate seeds
4 tablespoons sliced almonds
4 tablespoons Balsamic Herb Vinaigrette
(page 135)

1. Preheat the oven to 450°F. Line a baking sheet with parchment paper.

2. In a small bowl, toss the butternut squash with the oil, then spread the pieces on the prepared baking sheet. Bake for 20 minutes, or until soft and lightly browned. Let cool completely.

3. Meanwhile, prepare the quinoa. Place the quinoa in a fine-mesh sieve and rinse well with cool water to remove the bitter saponins. Drain well.

4. In a medium pot, combine the quinoa and stock. Bring to a boil, reduce the heat to low, and cover the pot. Cook for 15 minutes, or until the quinoa is cooked through. Let stand for 20 minutes, or until cooled completely.

5. Once cooled, layer the ingredients into 2 jars with tight-fitting lids, starting at the bottom and working up in this order: ½ cup butternut squash, ½ cup chickpeas, ½ cup quinoa, 1 cup kale, 2 tablespoons pomegranate seeds, 2 tablespoons sliced almonds. Close the lids tightly.

6. When ready to serve, add 2 tablespoons of the vinaigrette to the jars and gently shake to coat the ingredients with the dressing. Open and eat right out of the jar or pour onto a plate. This can be made up to 3 days in advance—just be sure to keep the vinaigrette separate until ready to eat.

GLUTEN FREE, NUT FREE *(replace almonds with peptias)*, VEGAN, DAIRY FREE

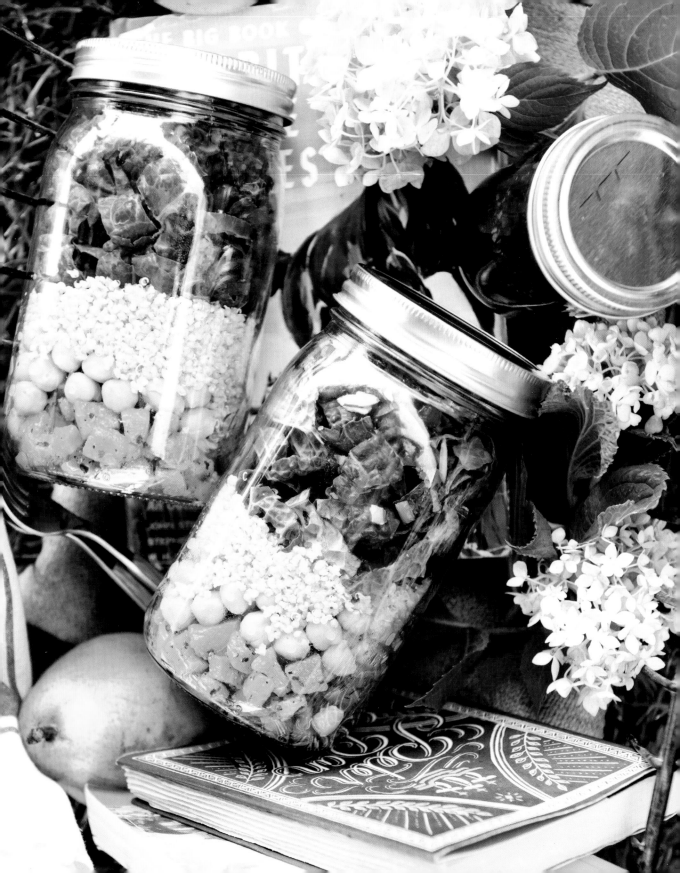

WALNUT LENTIL TACO MEAT

SERVES 2

¾ cups cooked brown lentils
⅓ cup walnuts, soaked in water overnight,
    drained and rinsed well
1 tablespoon tomato paste
2 garlic cloves, roughly chopped
1 teaspoon chili powder
½ teaspoon ground cumin
½ teaspoon paprika
¼ teaspoon sea salt
Pinch of ground red pepper

In a food processor fitted with the chopping
blade, combine the lentils, walnuts, tomato
paste, garlic, chili powder, cumin, paprika,
salt, and red pepper. Pulse until the mixture
resembles ground meat.

taco time salad

Mealtime can easily become taco time in my home—I love tacos! I occasionally talk myself into swapping the shell for a plate when a recipe turns out as good as this one. If you're craving tacos but trying to lighten up your diet, this recipe is for you. I like to make and store these in mason jars in my fridge so lunch is a quick grab and go. **SERVES 2**

1 cup Walnut Lentil Taco Meat (opposite)
1 cup cherry tomatoes, quartered
1 cup frozen organic corn kernels, defrosted
3 cups thinly chopped romaine lettuce

2 tablespoons thinly sliced scallions
1 ripe avocado, diced
4 tablespoons Cilantro Lime Dressing (below)

1. In 2 quart-size mason jars, layer the ingredients in the following order (from the bottom of the jar to the top): ½ cup taco meat, ½ cup cherry tomatoes, ½ cup corn, 1½ cups romaine, and 1 tablespoon scallions.

2. When you are ready to eat, add ½ diced avocado and 2 tablespoons of dressing to each jar, close the lid tightly, and gently turn the jar over to coat the other ingredients with the dressing. Open and enjoy!

CILANTRO LIME DRESSING MAKES ¾ CUP

¼ cup fresh lime juice
4 teaspoons honey
1 teaspoon ground cumin
½ teaspoon garlic powder

½ teaspoon sea salt
½ cup extra-virgin olive oil
2 tablespoons fresh cilantro, chopped

1. In a small jar with a tight-fitting lid, combine the lime juice, honey, cumin, garlic powder, and salt. Shake or stir until the honey is dissolved.

2. Add the oil, attach the lid, and shake vigorously until combined. Add the cilantro and shake one more time. Refrigerate until ready to use. Shake well before serving.

GLUTEN FREE, NUT FREE (*substitute sunflower seeds for walnuts*), VEGAN (*replace honey with maple syrup*), DAIRY FREE

sesame celery bowl

My dad is dedicated to eating a salad a day to keep the cancer away. He has courageously beat cancer twice with my encouraging mom right by his side and is doing all he can to keep it in remission. This salad is my personal take on the one that he makes daily, filled with alkalizing greens, natural fiber, plant-based protein, and healthy fats. **SERVES 2**

2 cups fresh spinach
1 can (15 ounces) chickpeas, rinsed and drained
2 ribs celery, very thinly sliced
2 carrots, shredded
½ cucumber, thinly sliced
2 scallions, thinly sliced
1 ripe avocado, diced
4 tablespoons sliced almonds
2 tablespoons Spicy Dressing (below)

Place 1 cup of spinach each in 2 bowls. To each bowl, add half of the chickpeas, celery, carrots, cucumber, scallions, and avocado. Sprinkle the sliced almonds on top. Drizzle 1 tablespoon of dressing over each bowl and serve.

SPICY DRESSING SERVES 2

1 tablespoon sesame oil
2 tablespoons rice vinegar
2 teaspoons tamari
½ teaspoon Sriracha
1 teaspoon pure maple syrup
2 teaspoons sesame seeds
1 garlic clove, minced

In a medium bowl, whisk together the oil, vinegar, tamari, Sriracha, maple syrup, sesame, and garlic until combined. Refrigerate until ready to use.

GLUTEN FREE, NUT FREE *(replace almonds with pepitas)*, VEGAN, DAIRY FREE

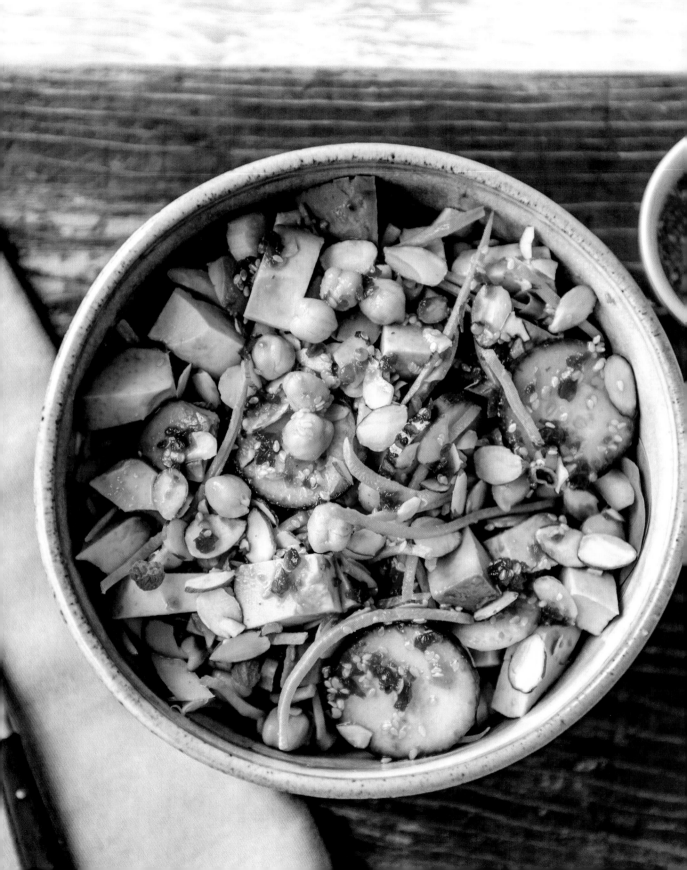

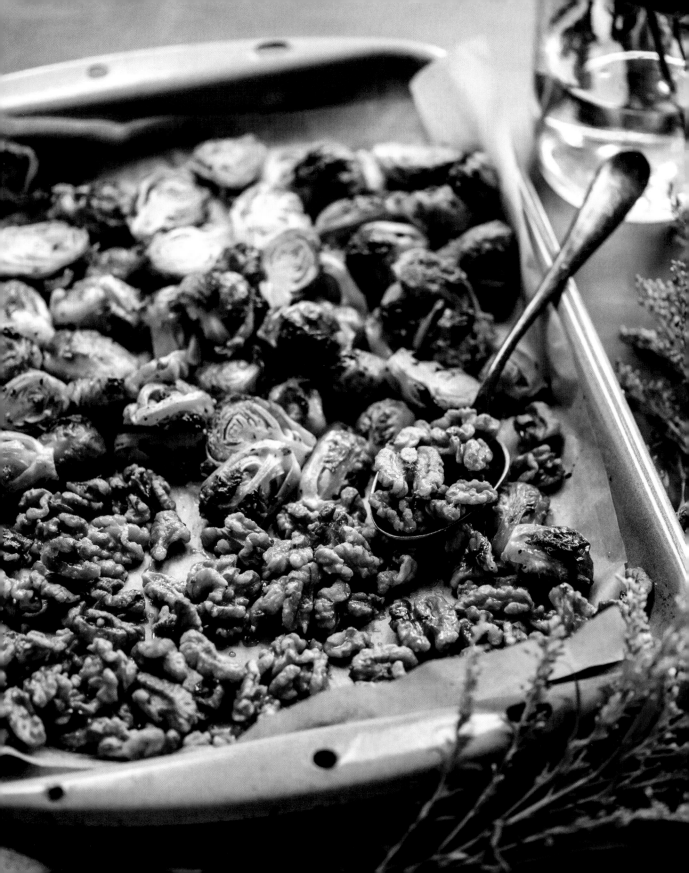

blackened sprouts

Brussels sprouts happen to be my favorite vegetable of all time. It started as a kid, when I would pretend they were baby cabbages for my Barbie doll. I would dip them in melted Velveeta cheese and devour them. Over the years, I have come to prefer my sprouts blackened and tossed with walnuts and maple syrup. **SERVES 4**

1 pound fresh Brussels sprouts, trimmed and halved
2 tablespoons avocado oil

Sea salt and ground black pepper
1 cup walnut halves
1 tablespoon pure maple syrup

1. Preheat oven to 425°F. Line a baking sheet with parchment paper, or grease it well.

2. In a medium bowl, toss the sprouts with the oil. Season well with salt and pepper to taste. Arrange in a single layer on the prepared baking sheet.

3. Roast for 20 minutes, or until the edges start to blacken.

4. Meanwhile, place the walnuts in a bowl and drizzle with the maple syrup. Toss until well coated. During the last 3 minutes of roasting time, place the coated walnuts on the same baking sheet as the sprouts to toast and caramelize.

5. Let cool slightly before serving.

GLUTEN FREE, NUT FREE *(remove the walnuts)*, VEGAN, DAIRY FREE

loaded frijoles

I love to season refried beans myself so I can have full control of the quality of the spices and the amount I use. If you want to kick up the heat in this recipe, feel free to add a pinch or two of ground red pepper. **SERVES 6**

1 tablespoon avocado oil
1 yellow onion, finely chopped
3 garlic cloves, minced
2 teaspoons chili powder

1 teaspoon ground cumin
2 cans (15 ounces each) pinto beans, undrained
¼ cup tomato sauce
Sea salt

1. In a 4-quart pan, warm the avocado oil over medium-high heat. Add the onion and sauté for 5 minutes.

2. Add the garlic and cook for 30 seconds, then add the chili powder and cumin and cook for 30 seconds.

3. Stir in the beans and tomato sauce. Taste and add salt, if needed.

4. Mash the beans, or puree them with an immersion blender, until the desired consistency is reached. Cook over medium-low heat for 15 minutes, or until the beans thicken. If the beans become too thick, add a little water.

5. Store in an airtight container in the fridge for up to 1 week or in the freezer for several months.

GLUTEN FREE, NUT FREE, VEGAN, DAIRY FREE

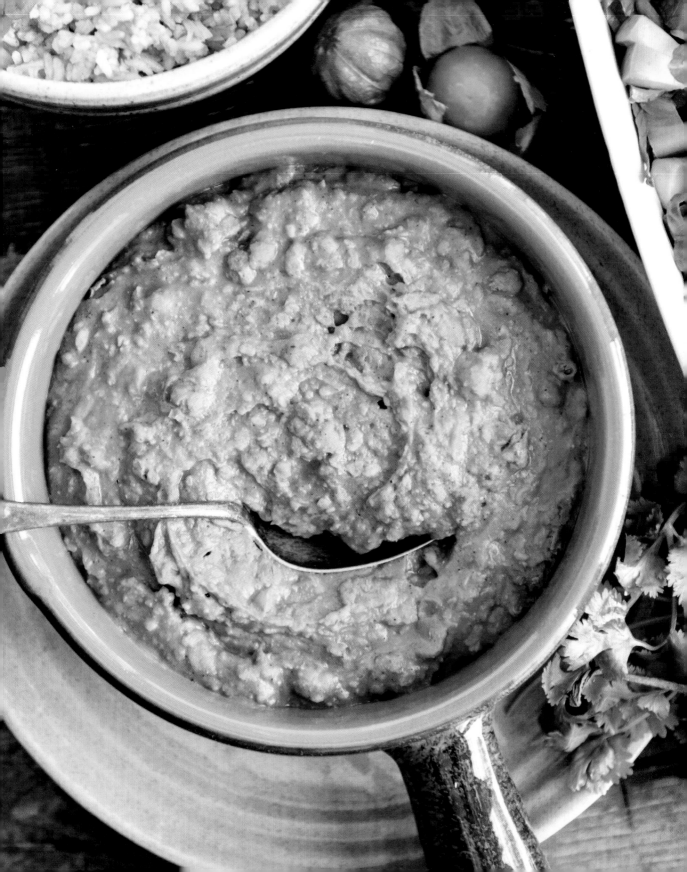

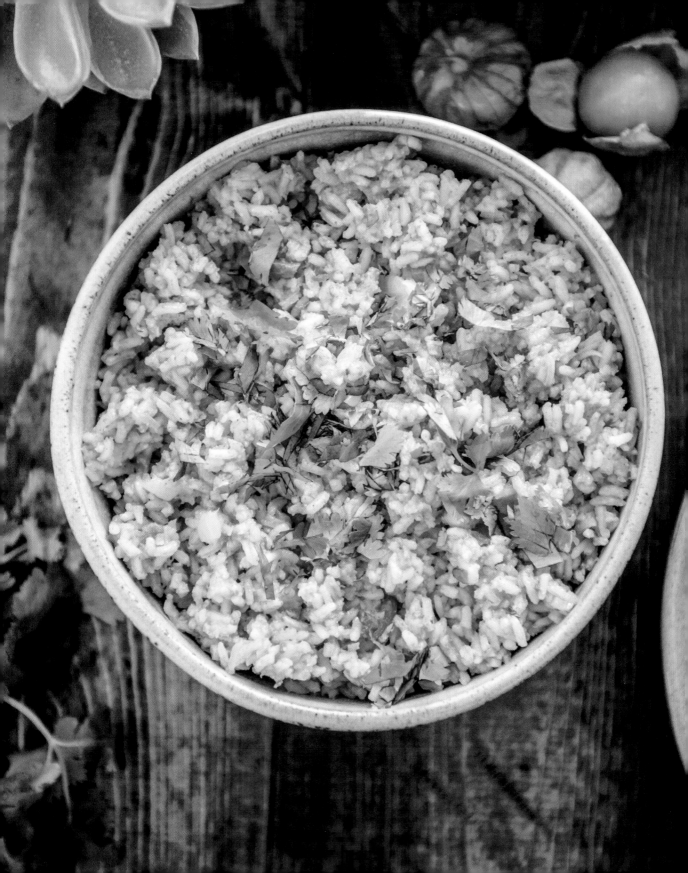

mexican red rice

The South has okra and sweet tea, like Los Angeles has rice and beans! You can't have one without the other. Born and raised in LA and now living in the South, I get the best of both worlds. This staple Southern California recipe goes nicely with the Loaded Frijoles (page 164), or it could be added to a salad for some extra sustenance. **SERVES 6**

2 tablespoons avocado oil
1 yellow onion, diced
2 cups white rice, long grain

3½ cups vegetable stock
1½ teaspoons sea salt
1 can (15 ounces) organic Mexican stewed tomatoes, undrained

1. Warm the oil in a lidded 4-quart pot set over medium-high heat. Add the onion and cook for 5 minutes, or until it begins to soften.

2. Add the rice and cook for 4 minutes, stirring constantly, or until the rice turns white. Reduce the heat as needed to prevent burning. This process converts the starch in the rice so that it doesn't get sticky or mushy during or after cooking.

3. Stir in the stock and salt, increase the heat to high, and bring to a rolling boil. Reduce the heat to low, cover the pan, and simmer for 10 minutes, or until the liquid is absorbed. The rice should still be firm.

4. Meanwhile, place the tomatoes and their juices in a food processor or blender. Pulse to chop, but don't puree.

5. Stir the tomatoes into the hot rice. Cover the pan and return it to low heat to finish cooking, 5 minutes. Let stand for 5 minutes before serving. In that time, the rice will soften more and absorb any extra liquid. Taste and add more salt, if needed.

GLUTEN FREE, NUT FREE, VEGAN, DAIRY FREE

cauliflower buffalo wings

I've never been a fan of chicken wings—yet I love the spicy-hot flavor! I was so excited when I got this plant-based recipe to work. **SERVES 4**

½ cup gluten-free all purpose flour
½ cup water
1 teaspoon garlic powder
½ teaspoon sea salt
1 head cauliflower, chopped

1 teaspoon virgin coconut oil, melted
⅔ cup Frank's RedHot sauce

FOR SERVING
Cashew Ranch Dipping Sauce (below)

1. Preheat the oven to 450°F. Line a rimmed baking sheet with parchment paper.

2. In a large mixing bowl, combine the flour, water, garlic powder, and salt. Whisk until smooth and well combined. Dip the cauliflower pieces in the batter, making sure each piece is well coated, and arrange on the prepared baking sheet. Bake for 15 minutes, turning the pieces over halfway through the baking time.

3. Meanwhile, in another large bowl, stir together the oil and hot sauce. When the cauliflower is done, transfer the pieces to the bowl with the sauce and toss well. Place the coated cauliflower back on the baking sheet and bake for 25 minutes, or until crispy. Let cool slightly. Serve the cauliflower with dipping sauce.

CASHEW RANCH DIPPING SAUCE MAKES ABOUT ½ CUP

½ cup raw cashews
4 teaspoons fresh lemon juice, divided
½ teaspoon dillweed

¼ teaspoon garlic powder
Pinch of paprika
Sea salt and ground black pepper

1. Place the cashews in a medium bowl. Pour 2 teaspoons of the lemon juice over the top. Add enough water to cover by a few inches. Let soak 2 hours, then drain and rinse well.

2. In a food processor, combine the cashews, ¼ cup water, dillweed, garlic powder, paprika, the remaining 2 teaspoons lemon juice, and salt and pepper to taste. Process until smooth and creamy. Scrape down the sides as needed. Store in the refrigerator until ready to use.

GLUTEN FREE, VEGAN, DAIRY FREE

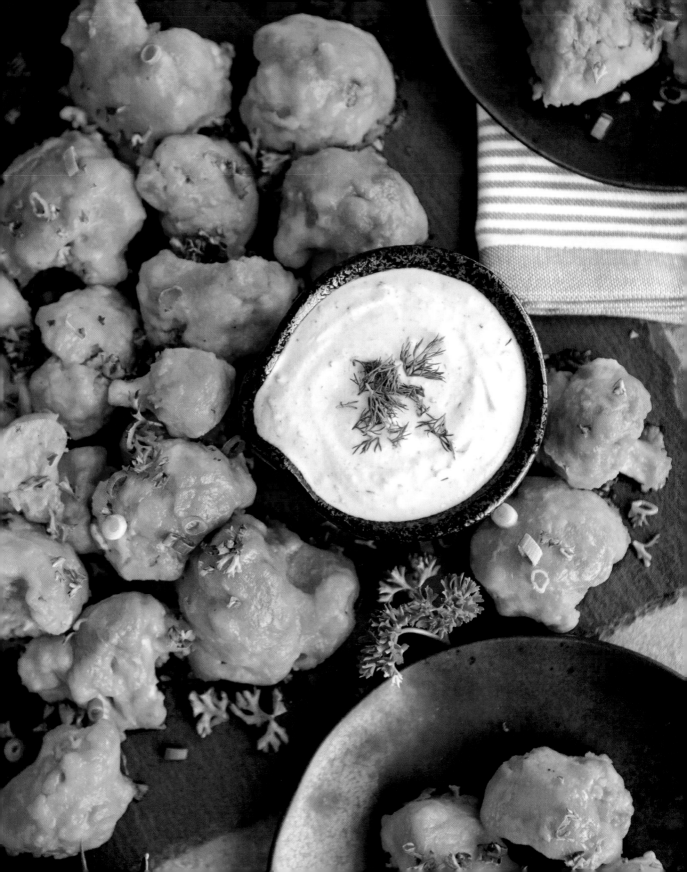

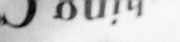

baked veggie fries

This side is an easy one to chop and prep for at the beginning of the week and just throw on a pan when you're ready for them. They make a great after-school or post-work snack and are amazing with the Everything Bagel Sprinkle. **SERVES 6**

2 cups fresh green beans, ends trimmed
1 carrot, cut into sticks
1 sweet potato, cut into sticks
2 tablespoons organic virgin coconut oil, melted

Sea salt

FOR SERVING
Everything Bagel Sprinkle (page 81)
Homemade Ketchup (below)

1. Adjust 2 oven racks so one is closer to the bottom of the oven and one is closer to the top. Preheat the oven to 425°F. Line 2 baking sheets with parchment paper.

2. In a medium bowl, toss the beans, carrot, and sweet potato with the oil. Arrange in single layers on the baking sheets. Sprinkle with salt to taste.

3. Bake for 15 minutes. Switch the baking sheets, top to bottom, and continue baking for 15 minutes longer, or until the fries are tender and golden on the edges. Season lightly with bagel sprinkle and serve with ketchup on the side.

HOMEMADE KETCHUP MAKES 2 CUPS

1 can (6 ounces) tomato paste
½ cup tomato sauce
½ cup diced yellow onion
½ cup apple cider vinegar
½ cup pure maple syrup
1 garlic clove, halved

½ teaspoon sea salt
¼ teaspoon ground cinnamon
¼ teaspoon mustard powder
⅛ teaspoon ground allspice
⅛ teaspoon ground nutmeg
Tiny pinch of ground cloves

1. In a saucepan, whisk together the tomato paste, tomato sauce, onion, vinegar, maple syrup, garlic, salt, cinnamon, mustard, allspice, nutmeg, and cloves. Bring to a simmer over low heat and cook for 30 to 45 minutes, or until the flavors blend.

2. Let cool slightly, then transfer to a blender and puree until very smooth. Pour into a jar with a tight-fitting lid and store in the refrigerator. It will keep for several weeks.

GLUTEN FREE, NUT FREE, VEGAN, DAIRY FREE

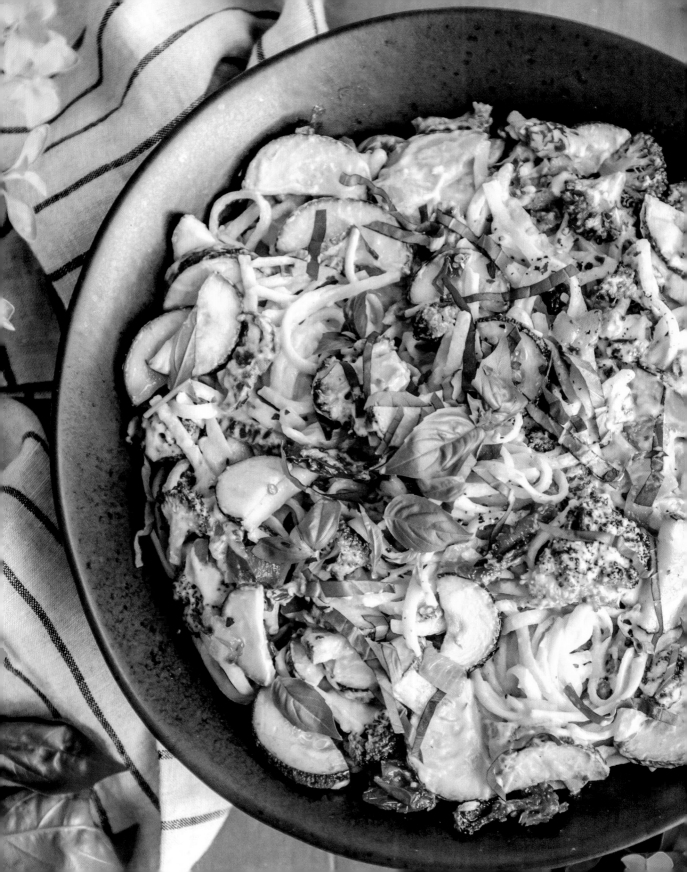

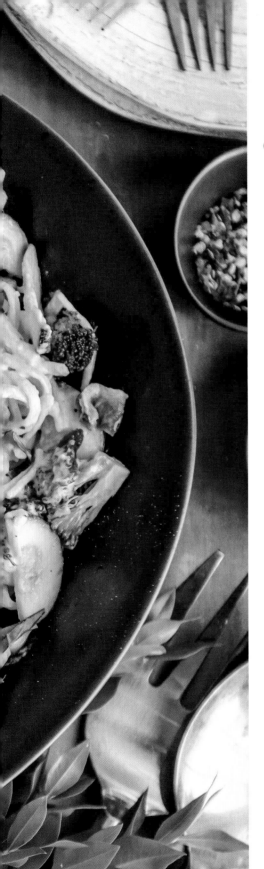

main dishes

savory quinoa pizza

A simple quinoa batter makes for a crispy-edged, tender, gluten-free pizza crust that takes almost no effort to make. These toppings are some of my favorites—especially the pesto—but feel free to top with whatever your heart (or tummy) desires. **SERVES 2**

FOR CRUST
1½ cups dry quinoa, soaked overnight in 6 cups water
2 teaspoons Italian seasoning or Italian Herb Blend (page 194)
1 teaspoon sea salt
1 garlic clove, finely minced
¼ cup avocado oil

FOR TOPPINGS
¾ cup Sun-Dried Tomato Pesto (page 72)
½ cup very thinly sliced fennel bulb
¼ cup thinly sliced red onion
1 cup baby arugula
1 teaspoon extra-virgin olive oil
Sea salt and ground black pepper

1. Preheat the oven to 450°F.

2. *To make the crust:* Drain the presoaked quinoa in a fine-mesh sieve and rinse. Transfer to a high-powered blender and add ¼ cup water, the seasoning, salt, and garlic. Puree, adding more water if needed, to make a very smooth batter.

3. Place a 12-inch cast-iron skillet or a rimmed pizza pan in the oven for 5 minutes. Add the avocado oil, return the pan to the oven, and heat for 5 minutes. Carefully remove the hot pan, and tilt it so the oil covers the bottom evenly. Carefully pour the batter into the center of the pan—don't pour too quickly or the oil could splatter. Spread the batter evenly. It should be ¼ to ½ inch thick, depending on the the pan. (If using a pizza pan, it may not reach all the way to the edges.)

4. Bake for 15 minutes, or until the top becomes somewhat dry and the edges golden. Carefully slide a large spatula under the crust to loosen it, then slowly flip it over, being careful not to splash any hot oil. Return to the oven and bake for 10 minutes.

5. *To top the pizza:* Carefully transfer the crust to a rack. Blot off the oil. Remove excess oil from the skillet or pan, leaving just enough to coat the bottom. Place the crust back in the pan and spread the pesto over the crust, then top evenly with the fennel and onion. Bake for 10 to 15 minutes to warm the toppings through.

6. Toss the arugula with the olive oil, salt, and pepper. Add to the top of the pizza, cut into wedges, and serve immediately.

- -

GLUTEN FREE, NUT FREE, VEGAN, DAIRY FREE

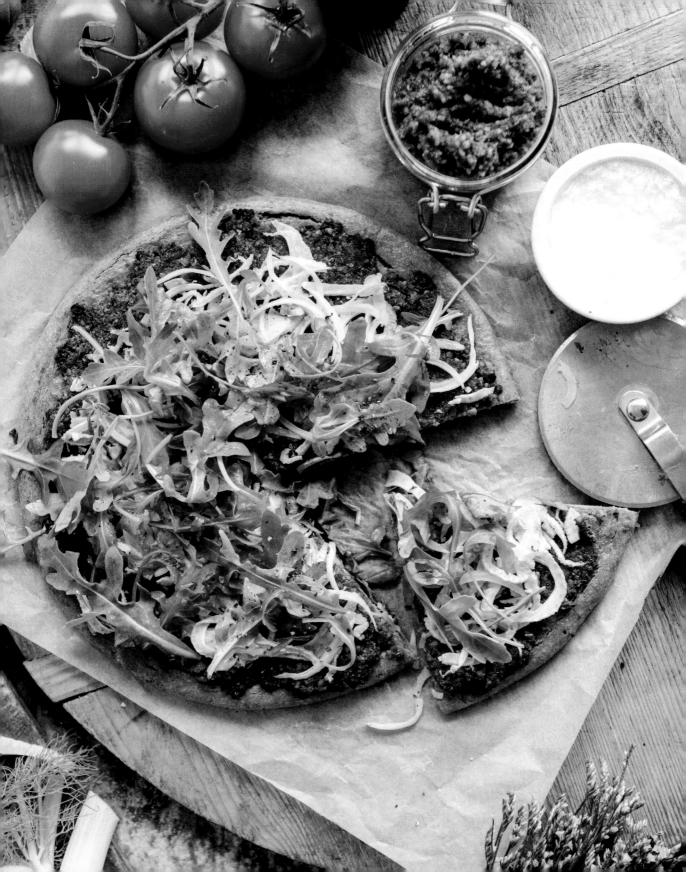

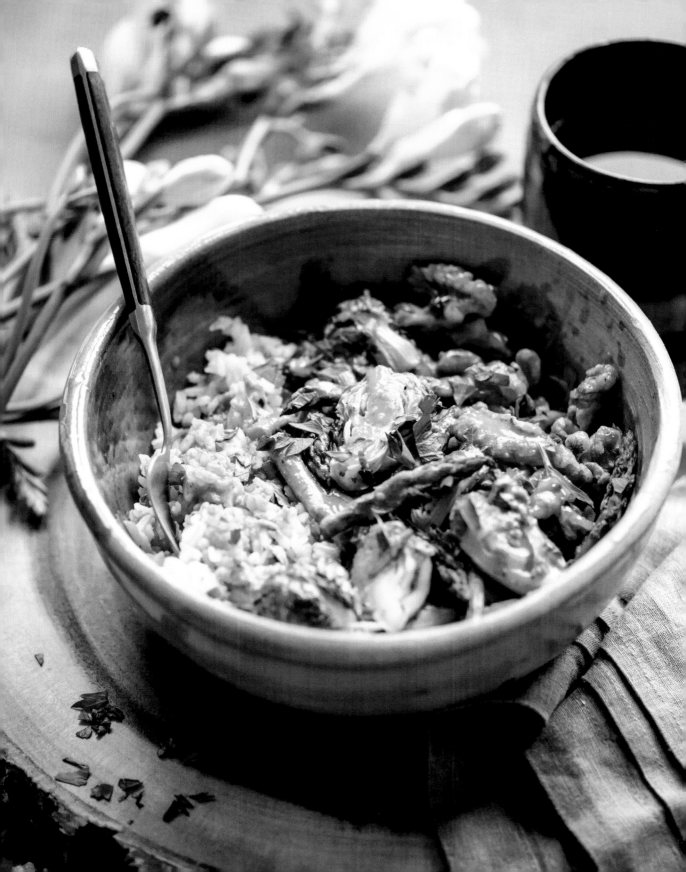

simple green veggie bowl

I often fly by the seat of my pants when it comes to dinner. I'll open the fridge and see what I can create out of the randomness—veggie bowls usually are the winner! I start the rice cooker while I decide what veggies to prepare. This dish is rich in carbohydrates, healthy fats, and plant-based protein—making it a balanced, awesome dinner for our family. The Coconut Sriracha Sauce kicks up the heat, but can be swapped with tamari to suit your taste preferences. **SERVES 4**

1 recipe Blackened Sprouts (page 163), partially prepared

1 pound asparagus, ends trimmed, cut into 2-inch pieces

2 tablespoons avocado oil

Sea salt and ground black pepper

FOR SERVING

3 cups cooked brown rice, warmed

Coconut Sriracha Sauce (page 61)

1. Preheat the oven to 425°F. Line a baking sheet with parchment paper.

2. Prepare the Blackened Sprouts recipe as directed and arrange the sprouts in a single layer on the prepared baking sheet. Roast for 10 minutes.

3. Meanwhile, toss the asparagus pieces with the avocado oil. Season well with salt and pepper. After the sprouts roast for the initial 10 minutes, move them to one side on the baking sheet and add the asparagus. Roast for 5 minutes.

4. While veggies are roasting, place the walnut halves in a bowl. Drizzle the maple syrup on top and stir to coat. Move the veggies again to one side on the baking sheet and add the coated walnuts. Roast for another 4 minutes or until the walnuts are toasted and caramelized.

5. To serve, spoon ¾ cup brown rice into four shallow bowls. Divide the veggies and walnuts between the bowls. Top with Coconut Sriracha Sauce and serve immediately.

GLUTEN FREE, NUT FREE *(replace walnuts with pepitas and modify sauce)*, VEGAN, DAIRY FREE

garden burgers

When I was 16, I remember swapping out a beef burger for a veggie burger and immediately regretting it: it was mushy, flavorless, and disgusting. Veggie burgers have come a *loooong* way since then—especially when you make them on your own! **SERVES 6**

1 cup gluten-free rolled oats
1 tablespoon avocado oil, plus more for cooking
1 yellow onion, diced
½ cup shredded carrots
4 garlic cloves, halved
1 can (15 ounces) black beans, drained and rinsed
½ cup fresh parsley, stems removed
½ cup sunflower seeds, toasted
¼ cup oil-packed sun-dried tomatoes, drained and chopped
1 teaspoon ground cumin

1 teaspoon paprika
1 teaspoon chili powder
¾ teaspoon sea salt
¼ teaspoon ground black pepper
¼ teaspoon ground red pepper

FOR SERVING
2 ripe avocados, sliced
1 ripe tomato, sliced
1 cup sprouts or microgreens
6 gluten-free or whole wheat buns, split in half and toasted, or 6 leaves romaine lettuce

1. In a food processor, pulse the oats until coarsely chopped. Set aside.

2. Heat 1 tablespoon oil in a skillet. Add the onion and carrots and cook for 10 minutes, or until softened. Add the garlic and cook for 30 seconds.

3. Transfer the onion mixture to the food processor with the oats. Add the beans and remaining ingredients. Pulse until everything is finely chopped and holds together but not pureed.

4. Line a baking sheet or plate with parchment paper. Form 6 equally sized patties that are about 4 inches in diameter and ½ inch thick. Cover the patties and refrigerate or freeze them until firm.

5. Heat a few tablespoons of oil in a nonstick skillet on medium-high heat. Place the patties in the pan, working in batches if needed. Cook for 5 minutes, then carefully flip. Cook for an additional 10 minutes, or until golden and crispy on the edges. (Frozen burgers will need a few extra minutes.) Serve with desired toppings on buns or as a lettuce wrap.

GLUTEN FREE, NUT FREE, VEGAN, DAIRY FREE

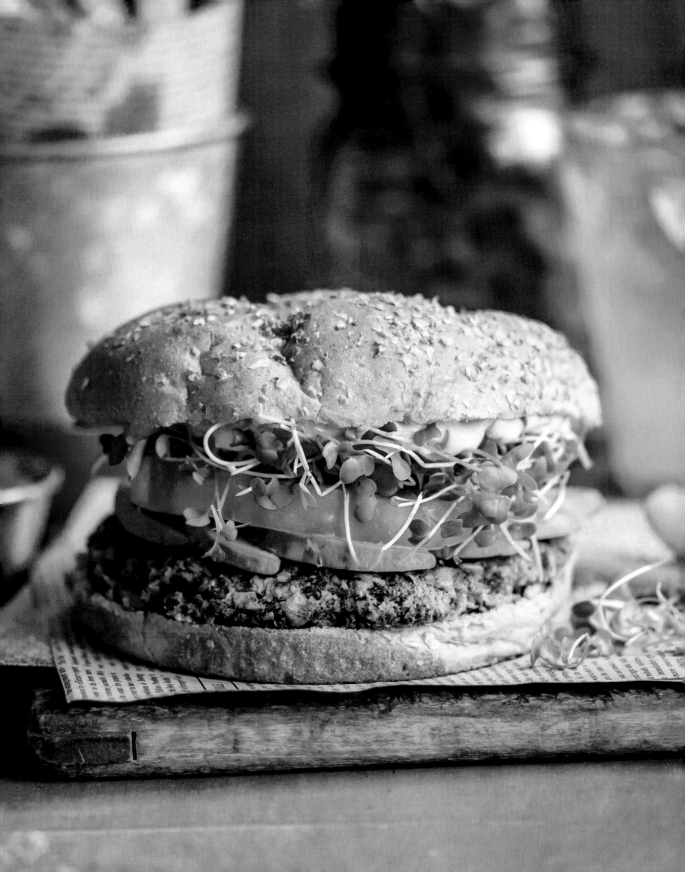

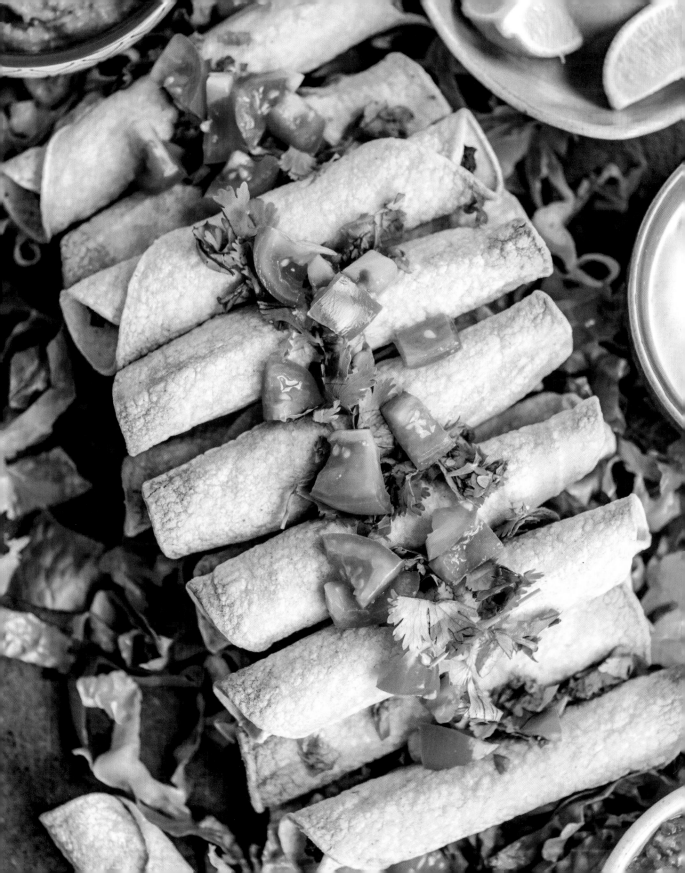

black bean little dippers

These are great to serve at parties. I like to make a double batch and freeze half for a future dinner—just remember to flash-freeze the dippers on a baking sheet before you fully freeze them so that they don't stick together. **SERVES 8 (3 DIPPERS EACH)**

Avocado oil, for brushing
1 yellow onion, quartered
1 poblano chile pepper, seeded and quartered
1 jalapeño chile pepper, halved and seeded
2 garlic cloves
1 can (15 ounces) black beans, drained and rinsed
½ cup fresh cilantro (leaves and tender stems), loosely packed

1 teaspoon chili powder
1 teaspoon ground cumin
1 teaspoon sea salt
24 organic corn tortillas

FOR DIPPING
Holy Guacamole (page 88)
Legit Salsa (page 91)
Cashew Cream (page 67)

1. Preheat the oven to 400°F. Line a baking sheet with parchment paper and brush with oil.

2. In a food processor fitted with the chopping blade, combine the onion, poblano pepper, jalapeño pepper, and garlic. Pulse 3 times to roughly chop. Add the black beans, cilantro, chili powder, cumin, and salt. Pulse 3 times, or until the mixture is finely chopped but not pureed. There should be a little bit of texture.

3. To prepare the dippers, work in batches. Place a few tortillas on a baking sheet and warm them in the oven for about 60 seconds, or until softened to prevent the tortillas from splitting during baking. Spoon a rounded tablespoon of the bean mixture down the center of each warmed tortilla. Bring one edge over the filling and tuck it in (like rolling a burrito with open ends) and tightly roll. Place the dippers, seam side down, on a plate until ready to bake.

4. Line up the dippers on the baking sheet, leaving a little space between them. Brush each one lightly with oil. Bake for 20 minutes, or until nicely browned. Serve with the dipping sauces on the side. Store leftovers in an airtight container in the fridge.

GLUTEN FREE, NUT FREE, VEGAN, DAIRY FREE

plant-powered cacao chili

Giving up meat can make a grown man cry . . . until he tries this chili. A hearty protein-packed chili is a staple dinner when autumn begins blowing cooler weather into town. Simmered to perfection with a variety of warming spices like cacao, cinnamon, and chili powder, this recipe makes even the biggest meat eater ask for seconds. Serve with Quinoa Corn Muffins, and he—or she—will ask for thirds. **SERVES 8**

1 tablespoon avocado oil
1 yellow onion, diced
1 green bell pepper, diced
1 jalapeño chile pepper, ribs and seeds removed, minced
4 garlic cloves, minced
¼ cup chili powder
1 tablespoon ground cumin
1 tablespoon cacao powder
¼ teaspoon ground cinnamon
1 can (28 ounces) organic crushed tomatoes, undrained
1 can (15 ounces) kidney beans, drained and rinsed
1 can (15 ounces) pinto beans, drained and rinsed

1 can (15 ounces) black beans, drained and rinsed
1 tablespoon pure maple syrup
½ cup water, for thinning (optional)
Sea salt and ground black pepper

FOR SERVING
1 cup Cashew Cream (page 67)
1 cup thinly sliced scallions
¼ cup thinly sliced jalapeño chile peppers
¼ cup fresh cilantro, chopped
2 ripe avocados, diced
2 limes, cut into wedges
Quinoa Corn Muffins (page 185)

1. In a 6-quart pot or Dutch oven, warm the oil over medium-high heat. Add the onion and bell pepper. Cook, stirring often, for 10 minutes, or until they start to soften.

2. Add the chile pepper and garlic and cook, stirring constantly, for 1 minute. Stir in the chili powder, cumin, cacao powder, and cinnamon, stirring for 1 minute, until the spices are toasted.

3. Add the tomatoes, beans, and maple syrup. Thin with the ½ cup water, if needed. Stir well. Reduce the heat to low and simmer for 45 minutes, or until the flavors blend. Taste and season well with salt and pepper.

4. To serve, ladle the chili into bowls and garnish with your choice of toppings and a muffin on the side.

GLUTEN FREE, NUT FREE *(skip the cashew cream)*, VEGAN, DAIRY FREE

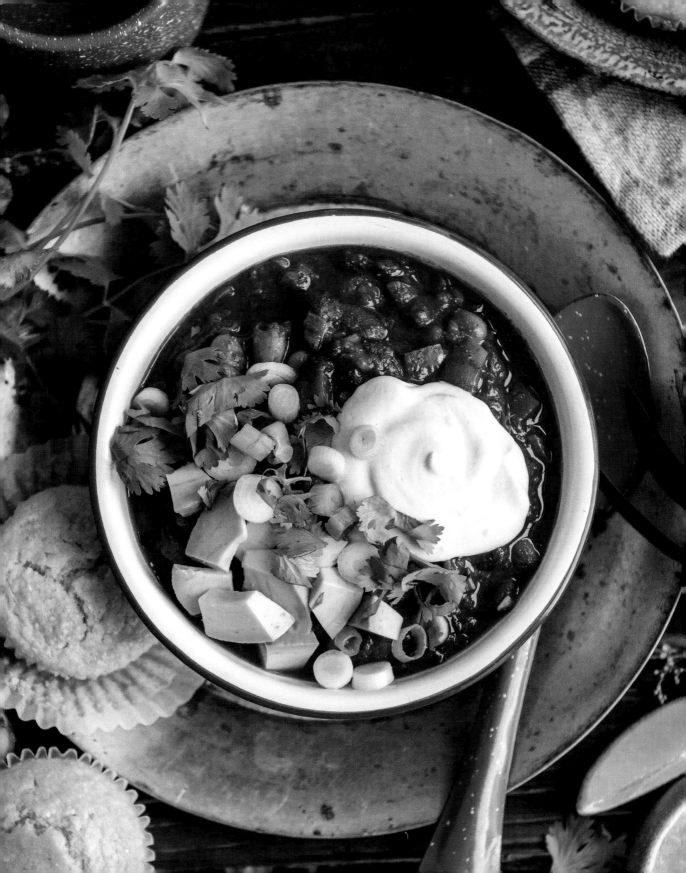

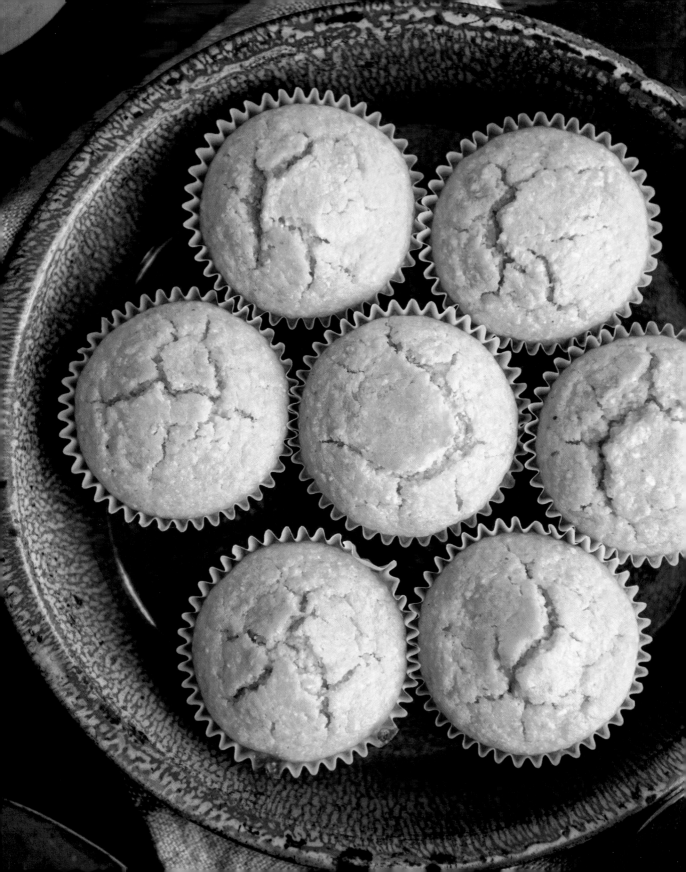

quinoa corn muffins

Moving to the South unlocked a whole new world of eating and drinking for me. From sweet tea to corn muffins to grits, I've come to love it all and have a hard time saying no to seconds. Well, these protein-enriched corn muffins are equally tempting—especially when dripping with honey. Save leftover quinoa from a dinner to use in this breakfast recipe.

MAKES 12 MUFFINS

¾ cup unbleached all-purpose flour
¾ cup organic stone-ground cornmeal
1 tablespoon baking powder
¾ teaspoon sea salt
¾ cup unsweetened plain almond milk
2 teaspoons apple cider vinegar
2 eggs

¼ cup honey
¾ cup cooked quinoa
½ cup organic virgin coconut oil, melted

SUGGESTED TOPPINGS
Strawberry Chia Jam (page 75)
Honey

1. Preheat the oven to 400°F. Line a standard muffin pan with paper liners.

2. In a large mixing bowl, whisk together the flour, cornmeal, baking powder, and salt.

3. In a large glass liquid measuring cup, stir together the almond milk and vinegar. Let stand for 4 minutes to curdle. Add the eggs and honey and whisk well.

4. Make a well in the center of the flour mixture. Add the almond milk mixture and stir just until moistened. Fold in the quinoa and oil. Scrape down the sides and bottom of the bowl to make sure the ingredients are incorporated, but don't overmix. The batter will be on the thinner side.

5. Fill the muffin cups three-quarters full. Bake for 20 to 25 minutes, or until the tops are nicely browned and spring back when lightly pressed. Serve the muffins warm or at room temperature.

- -

GLUTEN FREE *(replace flour with gluten-free all-purpose flour)*, NUT FREE, VEGAN *(replace eggs: 1 tablespoon ground flaxseed combined with 3 tablespoons water = 1 egg; replace ¼ cup honey with maple syrup)*, DAIRY FREE

three simple words led one passionate family

A few years ago, Ryan and I decided to focus on three words as a family, words that outlined our core values and shaped the kind of life we wanted to live. It wasn't easy picking those words, but once we said them out loud, they made my heart skip—seriously. It's amazing how powerful words can be! We call these words our family values: ADVENTURE, SIMPLICITY, and GENEROSITY.

We use these values like a compass when making family decisions. They guide us in deciding what to do when we aren't quite sure. For example: Where should we go on a vacation? What do we do when someone asks us to donate to a cause? What can we do to help that person in our lives who is in need? How do we live within our home?

It all falls back on our values. Here's how we put them into action:

ADVENTURE: We went to Guatemala with a team from our church and helped build a library and a home for a nonprofit that is passionate about educating and nourishing children. We flew to Cabo to house-sit for a friend and practice our Spanish. We snorkeled in Florida national parks and took an airboat ride through the Everglades.

SIMPLICITY: We cleaned out our home (even under the beds!), bought less, and simplified our space.

GENEROSITY: We gave more financially than we ever have before to so many wonderful people and organizations.

I don't say this to boast but to show you how impactful values can be to your family. I've never experienced so much awesomeness in one year—it was thrilling! We have to make space for the things that matter most to us: For every yes that year, there are five nos. But it is worth it, and I encourage you to get out there and live your values 100 percent.

What are your family's three words, and how can you bring them to life?

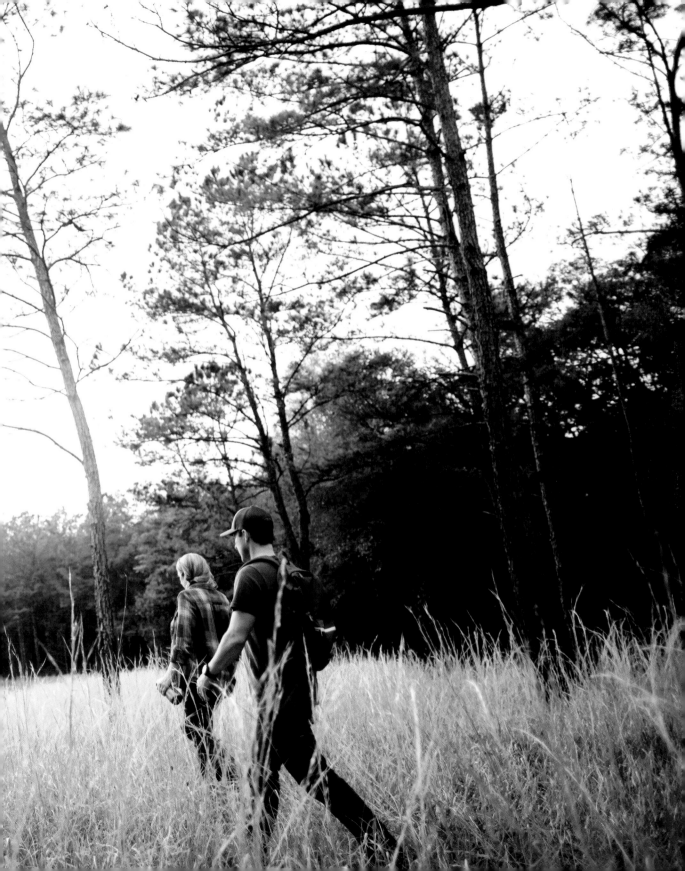

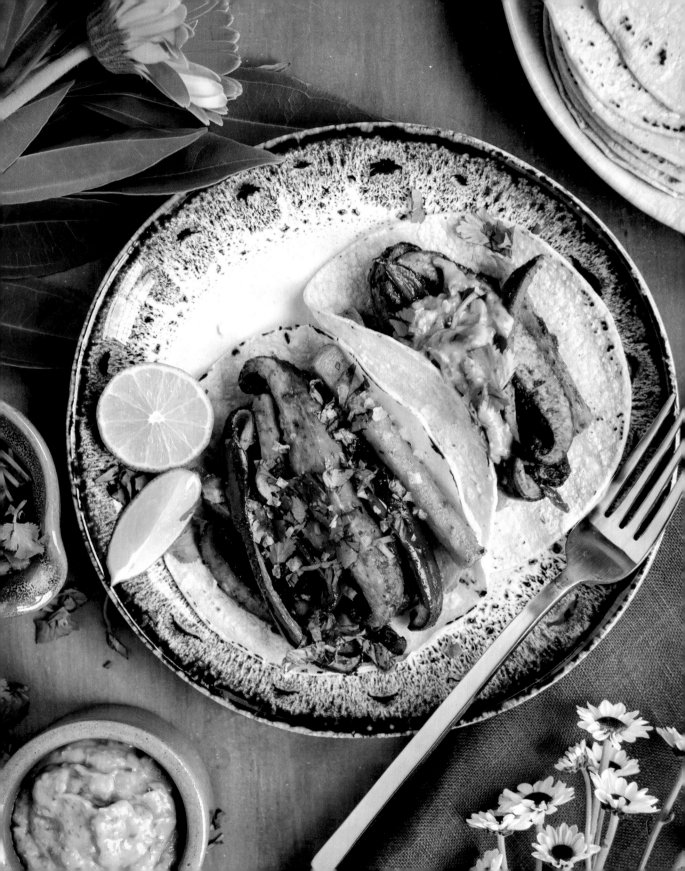

mushroom fajitas

When you start changing your diet to eat more plants, your world will be opened to so many new possibilities. Take mushrooms, for example. This used to be a "no, thank you" food for me, but now I find myself wondering, "What else can I make with mushrooms?" The best health benefits from mushrooms are achieved, however, when they are cooked to break down their cell walls, which are indigestible when raw. These fajitas are a great jumping-off point into the delicious world of mushrooms. **SERVES 4**

2 tablespoons fresh lime juice
2 tablespoons taco seasoning or
   Simple Taco Seasoning (page 107)
1 teaspoon pure maple syrup
2 to 3 tablespoons avocado oil
1 sweet potato, cut into strips
4 poblano chile peppers, seeded and cut
   into strips
1 yellow onion, halved and thinly sliced
   lengthwise

2 portobello mushrooms (6 ounces), cut
   into thick strips
Sea salt and ground black pepper

FOR SERVING
12 organic corn tortillas, warmed
Spicy Avocado Crema (page 206)
½ cup fresh cilantro, chopped
Fresh lime wedges

1. Preheat the oven to 450°F. Place a rimmed baking sheet in the oven to get very hot.

2. In a small bowl, combine the lime juice, taco seasoning, maple syrup, and 2 tablespoons oil and stir well.

3. In a large bowl, combine the sweet potato, chile peppers, and onion. Pour the lime juice mixture over the top. Toss well to coat. Add the mushrooms and toss again.

4. Carefully remove the baking sheet from the oven. Working quickly so the pan stays hot, drizzle a little oil over the pan and tilt to coat. Arrange the veggies in an even layer on the hot pan, season with salt and black pepper to taste, and roast for 20 minutes, or until the sweet potato is tender. (The other veggies will cook more quickly and become tender and blackened on the edges.)

5. To serve, spoon some of the filling into the warm tortillas. Top with a dollop of the crema and a sprinkling of the cilantro. Serve with lime wedges on the side.

GLUTEN FREE, NUT FREE, VEGAN, DAIRY FREE

veggie lentil stew

I was intimidated by lentils the first time I picked them up at Trader Joe's. I knew that there was a fine line between undercooking and overcooking, much like pasta. I don't have time to ruin a meal—I've got hungry mouths to feed! This recipe takes all that stress out, thanks to the slow-cooker method. **SERVES 8**

1 tablespoon organic virgin coconut oil
1 yellow onion, diced
¼ cup yellow Thai curry paste
1 can (13 ounces) full-fat coconut milk
2 cups dry red lentils, rinsed well and drained
2 carrots, peeled and diced
3 cups bite-size cauliflower florets
2 golden potatoes, cut into chunks

6–8 cups vegetable stock, divided
1 bunch kale, stems removed and roughly chopped
Sea salt

FOR SERVING
4 cups cooked brown rice (optional)
½ cup fresh cilantro, chopped
Crushed red-pepper flakes (optional)

1. Warm the oil in a large skillet set over medium-high heat. Add the onion and cook for 5 minutes, or until it starts to soften. Add the curry paste and cook, stirring constantly, for 2 minutes. Add the coconut milk, stir well, and bring to a simmer. Remove from the heat.

2. In a 6- to 7-quart slow cooker, combine the lentils, carrots, cauliflower, and potatoes. Pour in 6 cups of the stock, then add the onion mixture. Stir until well combined. Put on the lid and cook on low for 8 hours or high for 4 hours.

3. During the last 30 minutes of cooking time, stir in the kale. If the stew is thicker than desired, add more of the stock. Taste and add salt, if needed.

4. Ladle into bowls and serve with ½ cup of rice on top, if using. Sprinkle with cilantro and a pinch of red-pepper flakes, if desired.

GLUTEN FREE, NUT FREE, VEGAN, DAIRY FREE

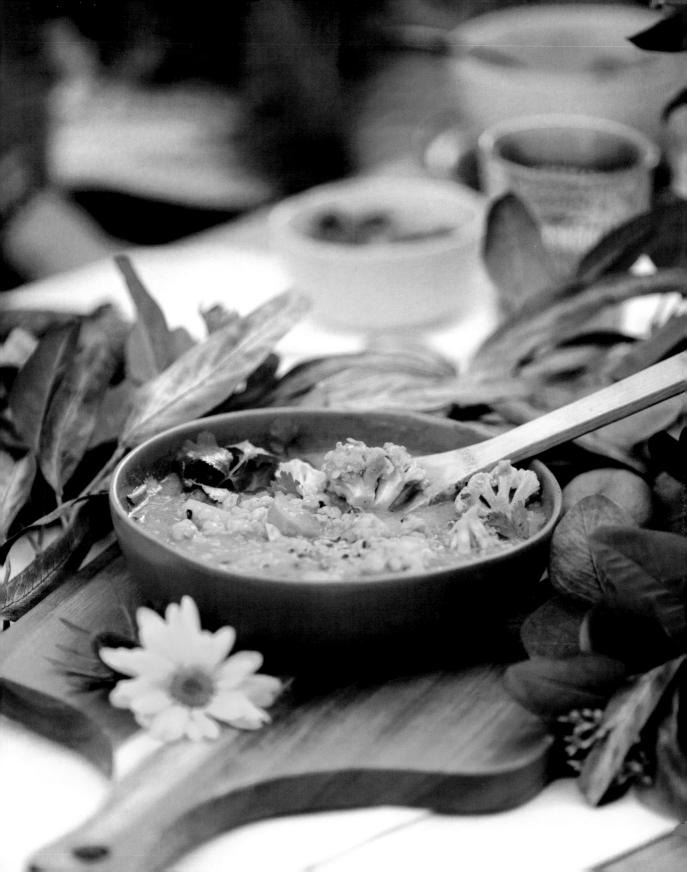

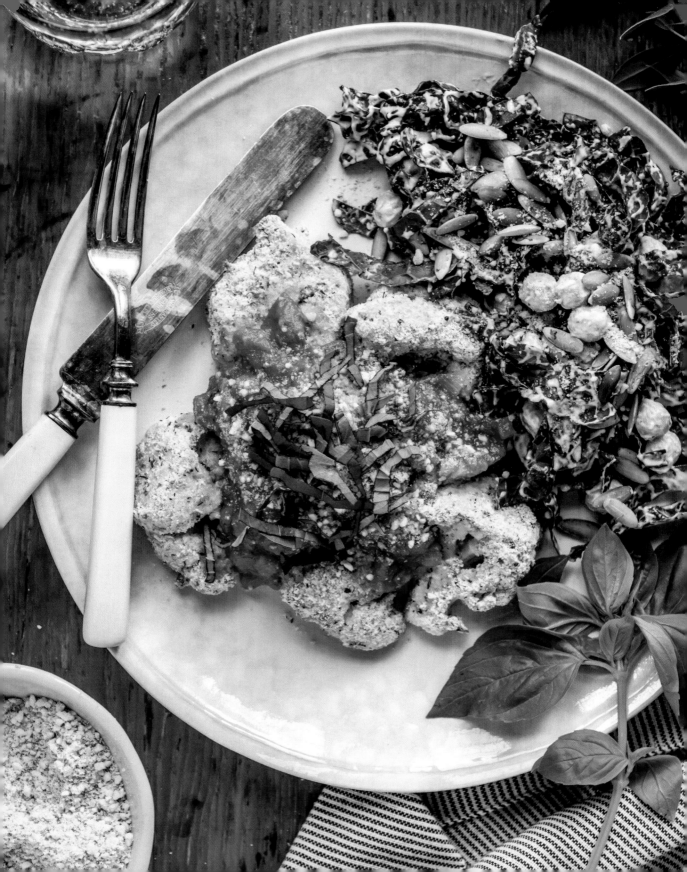

cauliflower "parmesan"

This plant-powered twist on an Italian classic is a great pre–race day meal. I used to carbo load with insane amounts of pasta and bread, but now I prefer to do it with cauliflower and kale, which is why I pair this dish with the Raw-ish Kale Caesar Salad (page 132). **SERVES 4**

2 eggs, lightly beaten
1 cup almond meal or almond flour
½ cup Cheeze Sprinkle (page 151)
1 tablespoon Italian seasoning or Italian Herb Blend (page 194)
¼ teaspoon sea salt

1 head cauliflower, cut into medium-size florets

FOR SERVING
2 cups Simple Marinara Sauce (page 194)
¼ cup Cheeze Sprinkle (page 151)

1. Preheat the oven to 425°F. Line a rimmed baking sheet with parchment paper.

2. Into a shallow bowl or plate, crack the eggs. Beat well with a fork. Set aside.

3. In another shallow dish, combine the almond meal, cheeze sprinkle, Italian seasoning, and salt.

4. Working with a few florets at a time, dip the cauliflower into the eggs to coat them well. Alternatively, dip a pastry brush into the eggs and brush over the entire surface of the florets.

5. Dip the coated florets into the almond meal mixture and press so the mixture adheres to the florets. Place on the prepared baking sheet. Repeat with the remaining florets.

6. Bake for 20 minutes, or until tender and golden.

7. To serve, transfer the florets to 4 plates. Top each with ½ cup of the marinara sauce and 1 tablespoon of the cheeze sprinkle.

GLUTEN FREE, NUT FREE *(replace the almond meal with whole wheat bread crumbs)*, DAIRY FREE

simple marinara sauce MAKES 4 CUPS

1 tablespoon avocado oil
1 yellow onion, diced
6 garlic cloves, minced
1 can (6 ounces) organic tomato paste
2 cans (28 ounces each) organic crushed tomatoes, undrained

1 can (15 ounces) organic tomato sauce
2 teaspoons Italian seasoning or Italian Herb Blend (below)
1 teaspoon pure maple syrup (optional)
Sea salt and ground black pepper
Pinch of crushed red-pepper flakes (optional)

1. In a 4-quart pot set over medium-high heat, warm the oil. Add the onion. Cook, stirring occasionally, until the onion starts to soften. Add the garlic and cook for 30 to 60 seconds, until fragrant.

2. Reduce the heat to medium, add the tomato paste, and cook, stirring constantly, for 30 to 60 seconds.

3. Add the crushed tomatoes, tomato sauce, Italian herbs, and maple syrup, if using. Cover and simmer for 20 to 30 minutes, or until the flavors blend.

4. If you prefer a smooth sauce, puree with an immersion blender or a traditional blender.

5. Season to taste with salt, black pepper, and red-pepper flakes, if using.

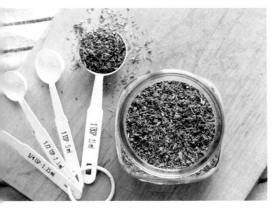

ITALIAN HERB BLEND MAKES ABOUT 1 CUP

¼ cup dried basil
2 tablespoons dried oregano
2 tablespoons dried marjoram

2 tablespoons dried rosemary
2 tablespoons dried thyme
2 tablespoons dried parsley
1 tablespoon garlic powder

In an 8-ounce mason jar with lid, combine the basil, oregano, marjoram, rosemary, thyme, parsley, and garlic powder. Attach the lid and shake well. Store in a cool, dry place.

GLUTEN FREE, NUT FREE, VEGAN, DAIRY FREE

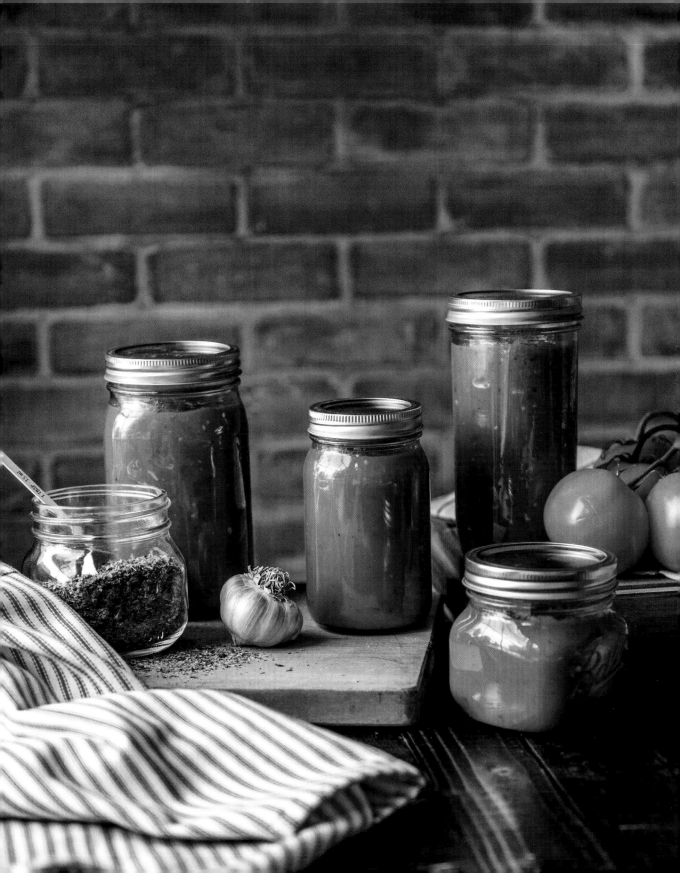

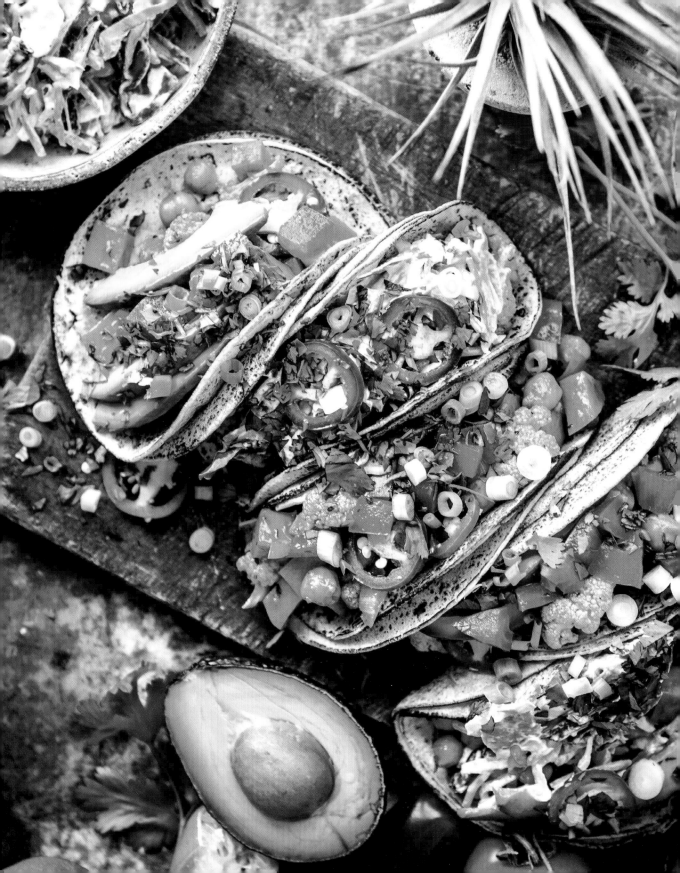

austinite tacos

Austin, Texas, is one of my favorite cities, thanks to the great music, the variety of healthy foods available, its natural landscape, and the fact that my awesome aunt and uncle live there. When I created this recipe, it just felt like it had an Austin flair going on, so I named it after that city. **SERVES 4**

1 head cauliflower, cut into small florets
1 sweet potato, cut into 1-inch cubes
1 yellow onion, diced
2 tablespoons organic virgin coconut oil, melted
Sea salt and ground black pepper
1 can (15 ounces) chickpeas, drained and rinsed
½ cup BBQ sauce, plus more for serving

FOR SERVING
12 organic corn tortillas, warmed
1 cup Simple Cashew Coleslaw (page 148)
½ cup fresh cilantro, chopped
Avocado slices
Sliced scallions
Diced tomatoes

1. Preheat the oven to 425°F. Line a baking sheet with parchment paper.

2. Spread the cauliflower, sweet potato, and onion on the prepared baking sheet. Drizzle with the oil and toss to coat. Season well with salt and pepper. Roast for 10 to 15 minutes.

3. Remove the pan from the oven and add the chickpeas. Drizzle the BBQ sauce over everything and toss to coat. Bake for 5 to 8 minutes, or until the veggies are tender.

4. To serve, spoon the BBQ filling into the tortillas and top each with a spoonful of the coleslaw, a sprinkling of cilantro, avocado slices, scallions, tomatoes, and any additional BBQ sauce you'd like. Serve immediately.

GLUTEN FREE, NUT FREE *(remove Simple Cashew Coleslaw)*, VEGAN, DAIRY FREE

almond butter swoodles

I remember the moment I took my first bite of this dish: My tastebuds rejoiced! It was everything I wanted, and then some. It's plant-based Asian fusion at its finest. **SERVES 4**

FOR ALMOND BUTTER SAUCE
¼ cup chopped yellow onion
1-inch piece fresh ginger, peeled and sliced
1 garlic clove
¾ cup almond butter
1 tablespoon tamari
1 tablespoon fresh lemon juice
1 tablespoon honey
1 teaspoon paprika
⅛ teaspoon ground red pepper (optional)

Sea salt and ground black pepper
¼ cup water

FOR SWOODLES
2 sweet potatoes, spiralized
¼ cup organic virgin coconut oil, melted
Sea salt and ground black pepper

FOR SERVING
½ cup thinly sliced scallions
½ cup fresh parsley, chopped
Simple Cashew Slaw (page 148)

1. Preheat the oven to 425°F. Line a rimmed baking sheet with parchment paper.

2. *To make the sauce:* In a food processor fitted with the chopping blade, combine the onion, ginger, and garlic and pulse a few times until finely chopped. Add the almond butter, tamari, lemon juice, honey, paprika, ground red pepper (if using), and salt and black pepper to taste. Process until combined. Stop to scrape down the sides.

3. With the motor running, pour the water through the feed hole. Keep processing until thick and creamy. Set aside.

4. *To make the swoodles:* In a medium bowl, toss the sweet potatoes with the oil, making sure the pieces are well coated. Place on the prepared baking sheet. The swoodles will overlap, but they will lose volume as they bake. Season lightly with salt and black pepper. Bake for 20 minutes, or until tender and golden. Check for doneness around the 10-minute mark, and check again periodically, to remove any swoodles that have cooked more quickly than the others.

5. Divide the swoodles between 4 plates. Top each serving with a little of the sauce, 1 tablespoon scallions, and 1 tablespoon parsley. Serve immediately with the cashew slaw on the side.

GLUTEN FREE, NUT FREE *(replace the almond butter with sunflower butter; omit the Simple Cashew Slaw)*, VEGAN, DAIRY FREE

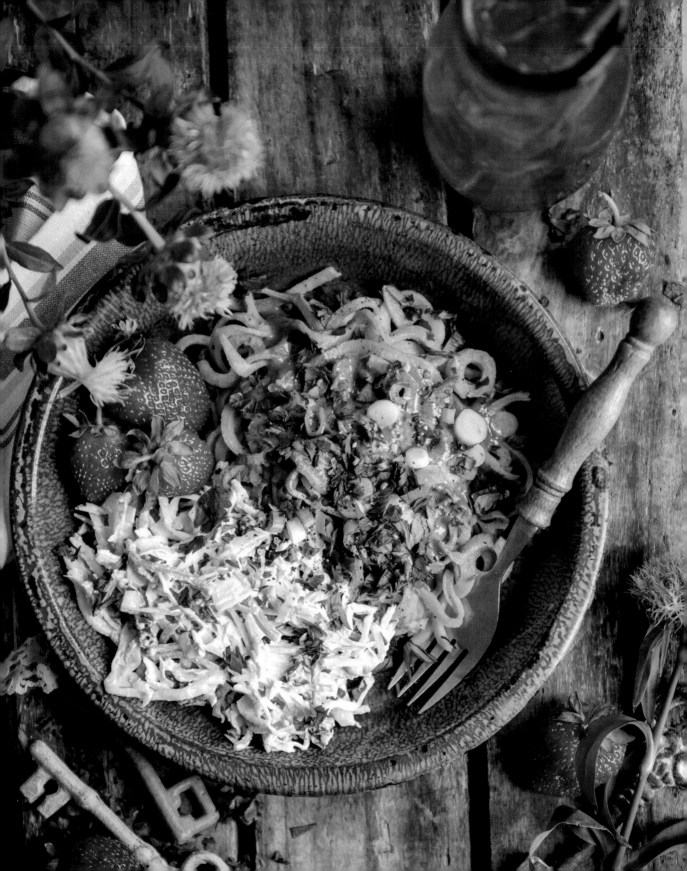

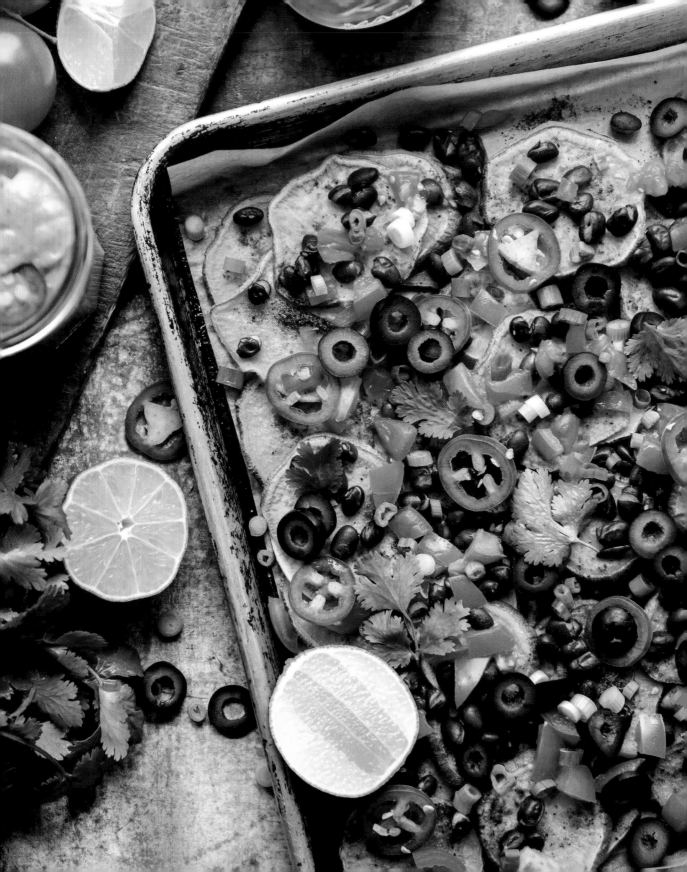

plant-powered nachos

This recipe can pull double duty as a delicious light dinner or a tasty appetizer. The seasoned sweet potatoes are baked until tender and then loaded up with our favorite toppings. Don't forget the Spicy Avocado Crema (page 206)—it's addictive! **SERVES 2**

2 sweet potatoes, thinly sliced into ⅛-inch rounds
2 tablespoons avocado oil
½ teaspoon ground cumin
½ teaspoon paprika
½ teaspoon chili powder
½ teaspoon garlic powder
½ teaspoon sea salt
1 cup canned black beans, drained

1 ripe tomato, diced
1 jalapeño chile pepper, thinly sliced
½ cup black olives, sliced
¼ cup thinly sliced scallions

FOR SERVING
½ cup fresh cilantro, chopped
½ cup Spicy Avocado Crema (page 206)
1 teaspoon Cheeze Sprinkle (page 151)

1. Preheat the oven to 450°F. Line a large rimmed baking sheet with parchment paper.

2. In a medium bowl, toss the sweet potatoes with the oil and arrange in an even layer on the baking sheet. The sweet potato rounds will overlap each other.

3. In a small bowl, combine the cumin, paprika, chili powder, garlic powder, and salt to make a seasoning mix. Sprinkle over the sweet potatoes.

4. Bake for 20 minutes, or until the sweet potatoes are tender and can easily be pierced with the tip of a sharp knife. Remove the pan from the oven and top the potatoes evenly with the black beans, tomato, chile pepper, olives, and scallions. Bake for 7 minutes, or until the toppings are warm.

5. Garnish with the cilantro. Serve with the crema and cheeze sprinkle on the side.

GLUTEN FREE, NUT FREE, VEGAN, DAIRY FREE

poblano enchiladas

Any chance I get to add veggies to a recipe without my kids turning up their noses, I take. These enchiladas are just that—packed with veggies and loaded with flavor. Loaded Frijoles (page 164) and Mexican Red Rice (page 167) make the perfect sides. **SERVES 6**

FOR SAUCE
1 jar (16 ounces) mild green salsa
½ cup canned full-fat coconut milk
2 teaspoons fresh lime juice
2 teaspoons ground cumin
½ teaspoon garlic powder
Pinch of ground red pepper, or to taste
Sea salt and ground black pepper
1 tablespoon arrowroot powder to taste

FOR FILLING
2 tablespoons avocado oil
2 golden potatoes, cut into ½-inch cubes

Sea salt
1 white onion, diced
2 poblano chile peppers, seeded and diced
3 garlic cloves, minced
1 bunch kale, stemmed and chopped
12 organic corn tortillas

FOR SERVING
1 cup shredded romaine lettuce
¼ cup pepitas
1 ripe avocado, sliced
Cherry tomatoes, sliced
½ cup Cashew Cream (page 67)

1. Preheat the oven to 400°F. Lightly grease a 13 × 9-inch baking dish.

2. *To make the sauce:* Stir together the sauce ingredients.

3. *To make the filling:* Heat a large skillet over medium-high heat. Add the oil for 20 to 30 seconds, or until shimmering. Add the potatoes and season with salt. Cook, turning the potatoes over every few minutes, until they start to soften and turn golden.

4. Add the onion and chile peppers to the potatoes. Continue cooking, turning the veggies periodically, until the onion starts to soften. Add the garlic, kale, and salt, and cook for 5 minutes. Remove from the heat. Taste and add more salt, if needed.

5. Wrap the tortilla stack in foil and place in the oven for 5 to 7 minutes.

6. Spoon one-third of the sauce onto the bottom of the baking dish. Fill each tortilla with ¼ cup of the filling and roll tightly. Place seam side down in the baking dish. Repeat with the remaining tortillas and filling. Pour the remaining sauce evenly over the top. Bake for 25 minutes, or until bubbling all over.

7. To serve, top with lettuce, pepitas, avocado, tomatoes, and cashew cream.

GLUTEN FREE, NUT FREE *(omit Cashew Cream)*, VEGAN, DAIRY FREE

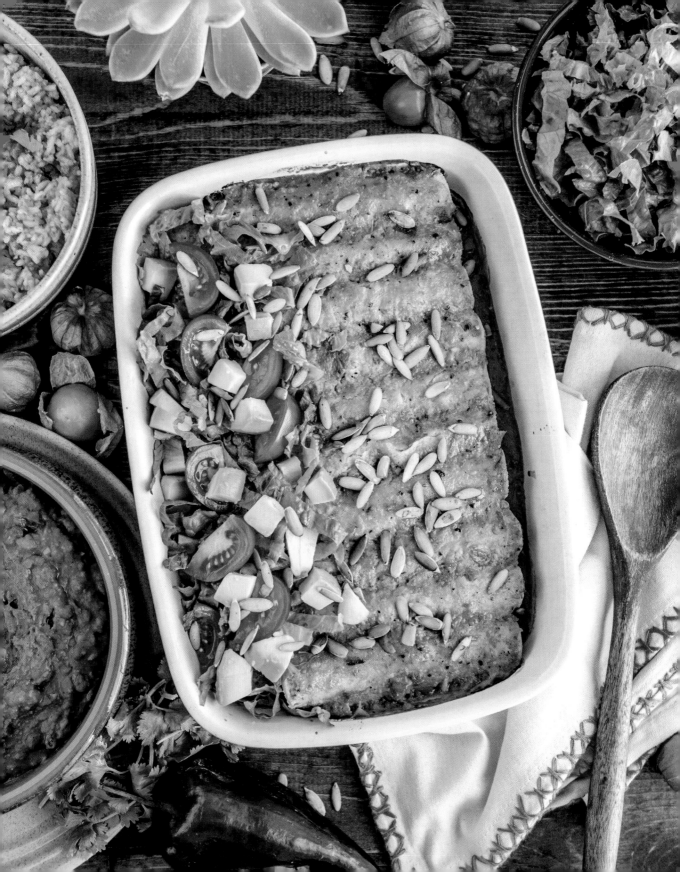

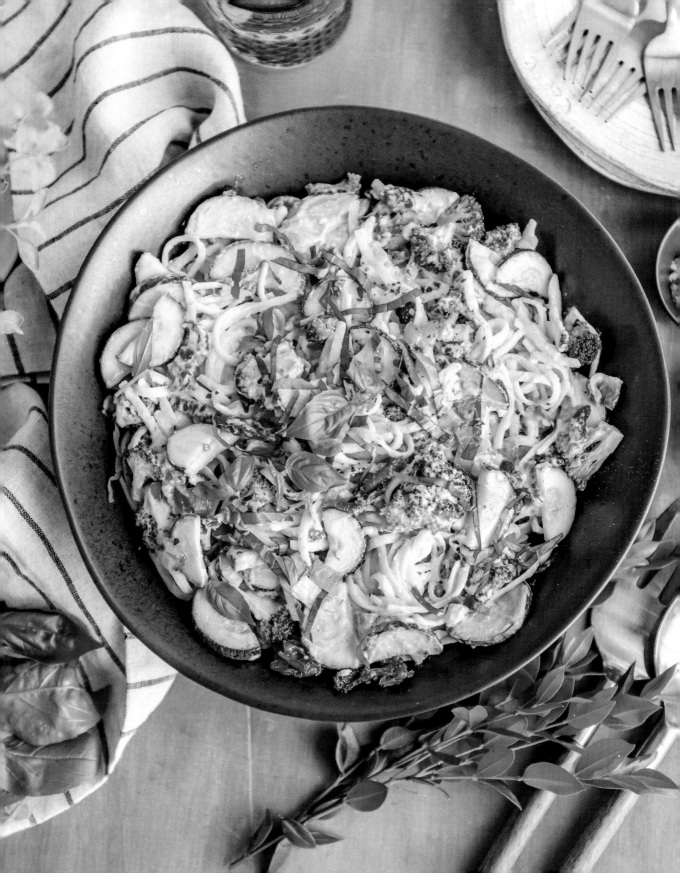

cauliflower alfredo

Traditionally, this type of meal is laden with dairy and would leave me hunched over in bed, feeling gross. Yet I would eat it over and over again because the taste was just too good to pass up. Well, this vegan rendition packs in the veggies and loads up on the sauce without the regret later on. *Mangia!* **SERVES 4**

FOR CAULIFLOWER ALFREDO SAUCE
1 tablespoon avocado oil
½ yellow onion, diced
2 garlic cloves, minced
2 cups cauliflower florets
½ cup unsweetened plain almond milk
2 tablespoons nutritional yeast
1½ tablespoons fresh lemon juice
1½ teaspoons miso paste
1 teaspoon Dijon mustard
Pinch of ground nutmeg
Sea salt and ground black pepper

FOR PASTA
8 ounces gluten-free fettuccini
1 tablespoon avocado oil
½ yellow onion, diced
Sea salt and ground black pepper
1 zucchini, halved lengthwise and cut into ¼-inch-thick half-moons
1 cup broccoli, cut into bite-size florets
½ cup sun-dried tomatoes, drained if packed in oil
½ cup fresh basil, cut into ribbons

1. *To prepare the sauce:* In an extra-large skillet, heat the oil over medium-high heat. Add half the onion and sauté for 5 minutes until it starts to soften. Add the garlic and cauliflower florets. Reduce heat to low and cook for 8 minutes, or until cauliflower is very tender. Transfer the cauliflower, onions, and garlic to a blender or food processor. Add the remaining sauce ingredients, and blend until smooth and creamy. Set aside until ready to use.

2. Cook the pasta in salted boiling water, undercooking it by a few minutes to prevent it from falling apart. Drain the pasta and rinse well to remove excess starch.

3. In the same extra-large skillet, heat the oil over medium-high heat and sauté the other half of the onion for 5 minutes, until it starts to soften. Add the zucchini and broccoli. Season with salt and pepper and sauté for 5 minutes until tender-crisp. Add the tomatoes, the reserved Alfredo sauce, and the pasta, and heat gently for 3 minutes.

4. To serve, spoon into bowls and top with fresh basil. Serve immediately.

GLUTEN FREE, NUT FREE *(replace almond milk with unsweetened plain coconut milk)*, VEGAN, DAIRY FREE

spicy avocado crema

Think of this as a guacamole dressing—thick, creamy, with a hint of spice and fresh lime juice. Coconut milk gives it a nice drizzling quality. You can dip taquitos in it or cover your salad with it. So many uses! Feel free to add more spice if you can take the heat. **MAKES ABOUT ¾ CUP**

1 ripe avocado, halved and pitted
¼ cup canned full-fat coconut milk
2 tablespoons fresh lime juice

½ seranno chile pepper, seeds and ribs removed
¼ cup fresh cilantro, chopped
¼ teaspoon sea salt

1. In a blender or food processor, combine the avocado, coconut milk, lime juice, chile pepper, cilantro, and salt.

2. Blend or process until smooth. Taste and add more salt or lime juice if needed. Transfer to an airtight container and refrigerate until ready to use.

GLUTEN FREE, NUT FREE, VEGAN, DAIRY FREE

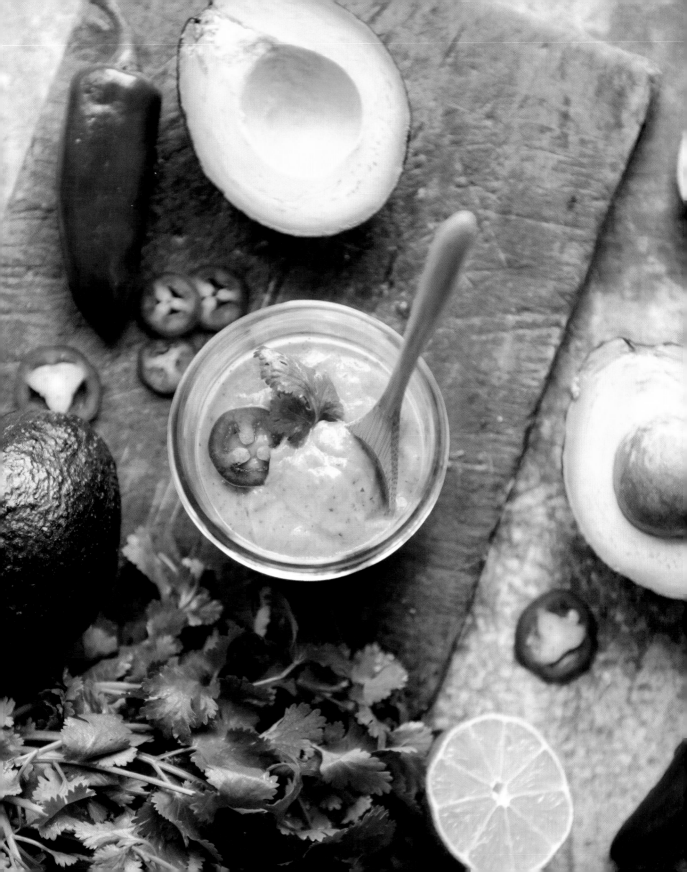

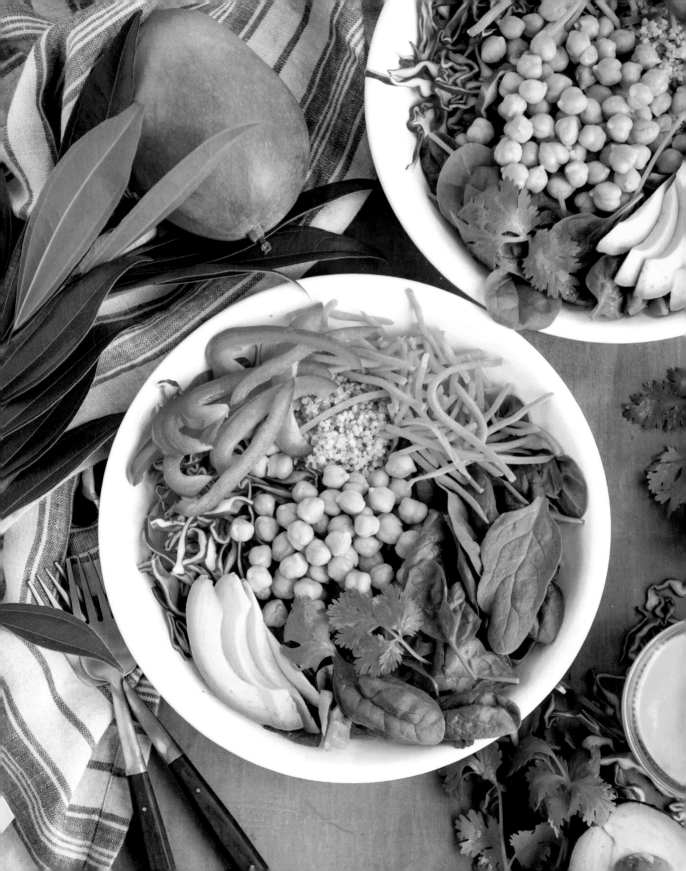

mango chickpea bowls

There are certain ingredients that fuse together like magic—and this bowl is all about that. It's got a little bit of everything: crunch, cream, bite, sweetness, and heat. If you're not a fan of cilantro, you can easily swap it out for another fresh herb like parsley or basil. **SERVES 4**

1 cup white or red dry quinoa
2 cups vegetable stock
2 cups fresh spinach
2 cups grated or finely shredded red cabbage
1 can (15 ounces) chickpeas, drained and rinsed

1 ripe avocado, thinly sliced
1 red bell pepper, thinly sliced
1 cup shredded carrots
4 tablespoons Mango-Ginger-Turmeric Sauce (below)
½ cup fresh cilantro, chopped

1. If the quinoa is not prerinsed (check the package), place it in a fine-mesh sieve and rinse well with cool water to remove the bitter saponins on the quinoa. Drain well.

2. In a saucepan, combine the quinoa and stock. Bring to a boil, then reduce the heat to low, cover, and cook for 15 minutes, or until the quinoa is cooked through. Let stand for 5 minutes.

3. Into each of 4 shallow serving bowls, place ½ cup spinach, ½ cup cabbage, and ½ cup quinoa. Spoon ½ cup chickpeas into the center of each. Arrange one-quarter of the avocado, bell pepper, and carrots on top of each bowl. Spoon 1 tablespoon of the mango sauce on top of each veggie bowl, sprinkle with the cilantro, and serve.

MANGO-GINGER-TURMERIC SAUCE SERVES 4

1 mango, diced
¼ cup fresh lime juice
2 tablespoons extra-virgin olive oil
1 teaspoon pure maple syrup

1 teaspoon finely minced fresh ginger
½ teaspoon ground turmeric
¼ teaspoon sea salt
Pinch of ground red pepper

In a blender or food processor, combine the mango, lime juice, oil, maple syrup, ginger, turmeric, salt, and red pepper and puree until smooth. Set aside if using immediately, or refrigerate until ready to use later.

GLUTEN FREE, NUT FREE, VEGAN, DAIRY FREE

thai lettuce wraps

When I became a vegetarian at 16 years old, one of the meals I missed the most was the chicken lettuce wraps from my fav Chinese restaurant. Then a vegetarian version came out on the market, and I was rejoicing—that is, until I learned that version contains gluten, which just seems strange. This recipe is inspired by those, yet this dish adds a lot more nourishment and flavors to make me one happy gluten-free vegetarian. **SERVES 4**

2 tablespoons organic virgin coconut oil
1 rib celery, thinly sliced
¼ cup minced shallots
1 tablespoon minced fresh ginger
3 garlic cloves, minced
8 ounces baby bella or white button mushrooms, finely chopped
2 heaping cups walnuts, chopped
2 tablespoons fresh lime juice
2 tablespoons tamari
2 tablespoons coconut sugar

1 tablespoon rice vinegar
2 tablespoons fresh mint, chopped
2 tablespoons fresh cilantro, chopped
Pinch of crushed red-pepper flakes

FOR SERVING
12 leaves butter lettuce
1 cup shredded carrots
½ cup raw cashews, chopped
¼ cup fresh cilantro, chopped
¼ cup thinly sliced scallions
Lime wedges

1. Warm a large skillet over medium-high heat. Add the oil and heat until shimmering. Add the celery and shallots and cook for 5 minutes. Add the ginger and garlic and cook for 1 minute.

2. Stir in the mushrooms. Cook, stirring occasionally, until the mushrooms release their liquid and it evaporates, and the mushrooms start to brown nicely. Add the walnuts and cook for 1 to 2 minutes to toast them.

3. Stir in the lime juice, tamari, coconut sugar, and rice vinegar. Simmer for 15 minutes, or until the sauce thickens slightly. Remove from the heat and stir in the mint, cilantro, and red-pepper flakes. Taste and add more tamari, if desired, for more saltiness. Keep warm until ready to serve.

4. To serve, spoon some of the vegetables into the lettuce leaves. Top with a sprinkling of carrots, cashews, cilantro, and scallions and add a squeeze of lime. Serve warm.

GLUTEN FREE, NUT FREE *(remove walnuts and double mushrooms, remove cashews)*, VEGAN, DAIRY FREE

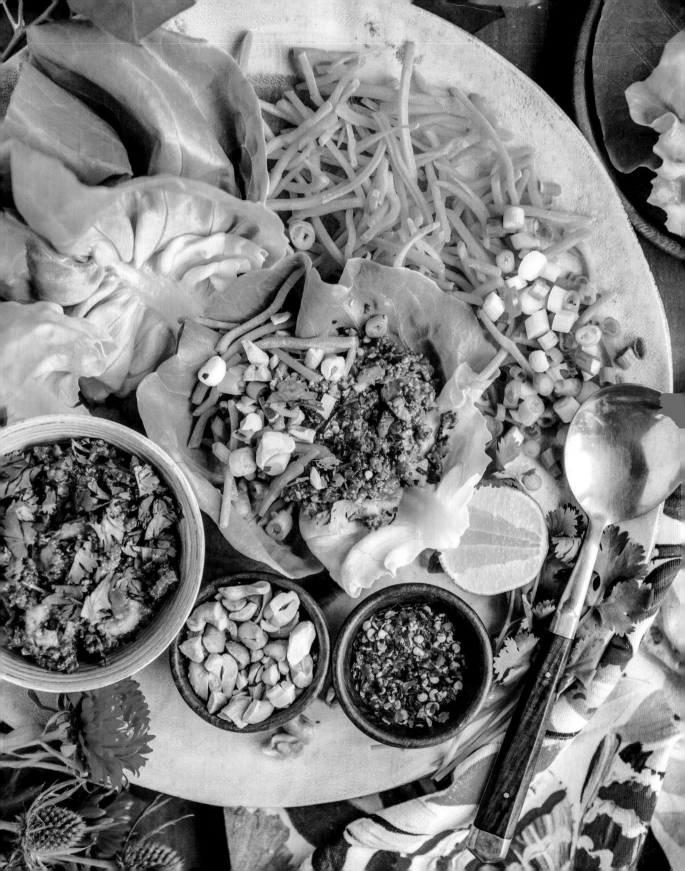

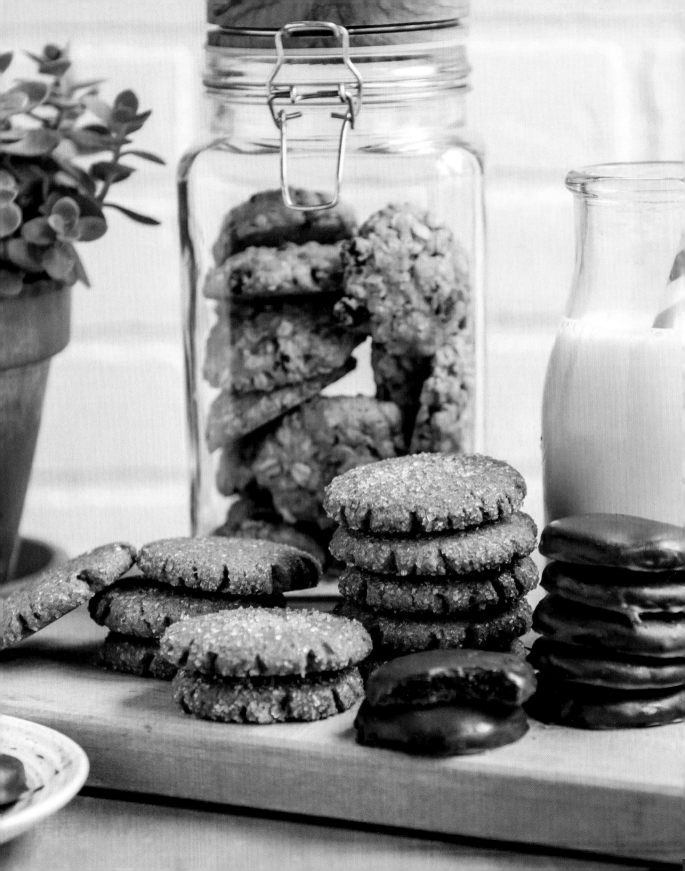

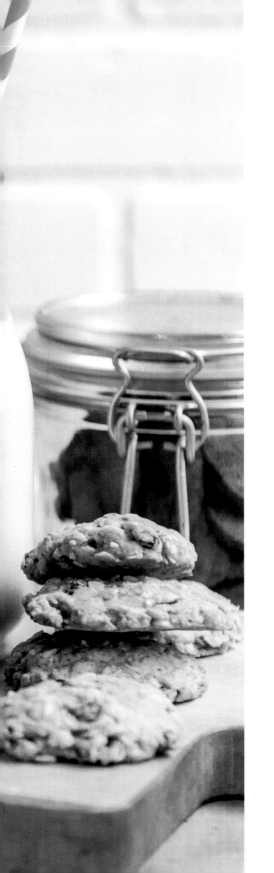

desserts

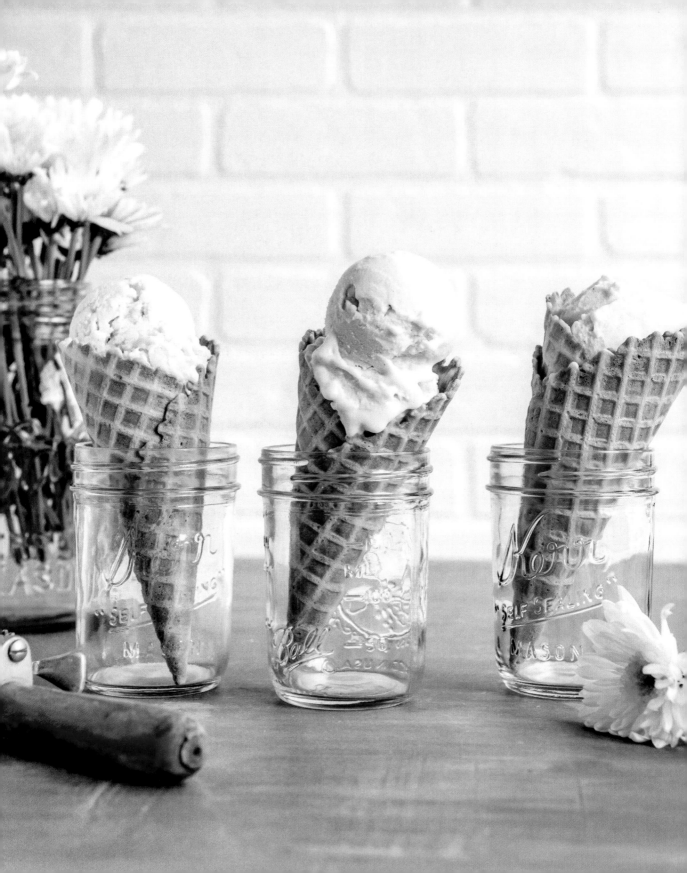

vanilla bean ice cream

This dairy-free ice cream is full of healthy plant-based fats and natural sweeteners, making it a nourishing and satisfying dessert. You'll need an ice cream maker to get the ideal consistency. **MAKES ABOUT 1 QUART**

2 cans (13 ounces each) full-fat coconut milk, at room temperature
½ cup organic sugar
1 tablespoon pure maple syrup

1 vanilla bean, split lengthwise and seeds scraped out
1 tablespoon arrowroot powder
Pinch of sea salt

1. Shake the cans of coconut milk before opening. Open and reserve ¼ cup of the milk. Pour the remainder into a 3-quart saucepan. Whisk in the sugar and maple syrup. Heat gently over medium heat until very hot, being careful not to let the mixture reach a boil. (Boiling will cause the coconut milk to separate, and the mixture will become oily.) Add the vanilla bean and seeds.

2. Meanwhile, in a small bowl, stir together the reserved ¼ cup coconut milk and the arrowroot powder and salt to make a slurry. (This will thicken the ice cream base.) If the mixture is lumpy, keep stirring and press the lumps against the bowl with the back of a spoon to help dissolve them.

3. Pour the arrowroot mixture into the pan with the coconut milk mixture, whisking continuously. Cook for 5 to 7 minutes—not letting it boil—until thickened. It should coat the back of a wooden spoon or be the texture of thin yogurt. Pour into a clean bowl. Remove the vanilla bean, scraping any seeds or pulp still attached to the bean back into the bowl. Let the mixture cool, then refrigerate for several hours or overnight, until very cold.

4. Churn the mixture in an ice cream maker, following the manufacturer's directions. Transfer the ice cream to an airtight freezer container and chill until firm.

GLUTEN FREE, NUT FREE, VEGAN, DAIRY FREE

mango-peach sorbet

Did you know that a high-powered blender can double as an ice cream maker? It's true! We love the bright flavors of mango and peach blended together for a creamy, naturally sweetened frozen dessert. PS: A scoop or two of sorbet + fizzy water = a real treat! **SERVES 4**

2 cups frozen mango
2 cups frozen peaches

1 cup fresh orange juice
Pure maple syrup (optional)

1. In a high-powered blender, combine the mango, peaches, and orange juice. Puree, stopping to scrape down the sides as needed. Add a little extra liquid if the blender is struggling. Taste; add maple syrup if the mixture needs sweetening.

2. Serve immediately for soft serve sorbet, or, for scoopable sorbet, transfer to an airtight container and freeze until firm enough to scoop. Store leftovers in the freezer.

GLUTEN FREE, NUT FREE, VEGAN, DAIRY FREE

rawkstar tip

Other fruit can be substituted for the mango and peaches. Depending on the type of fruit used and the level of ripeness and sweetness, the sorbet may or may not need extra sweetener. Water or another fresh squeezed or no-sugar-added fruit juice can be substituted for the orange juice, or two peeled oranges can also be used.

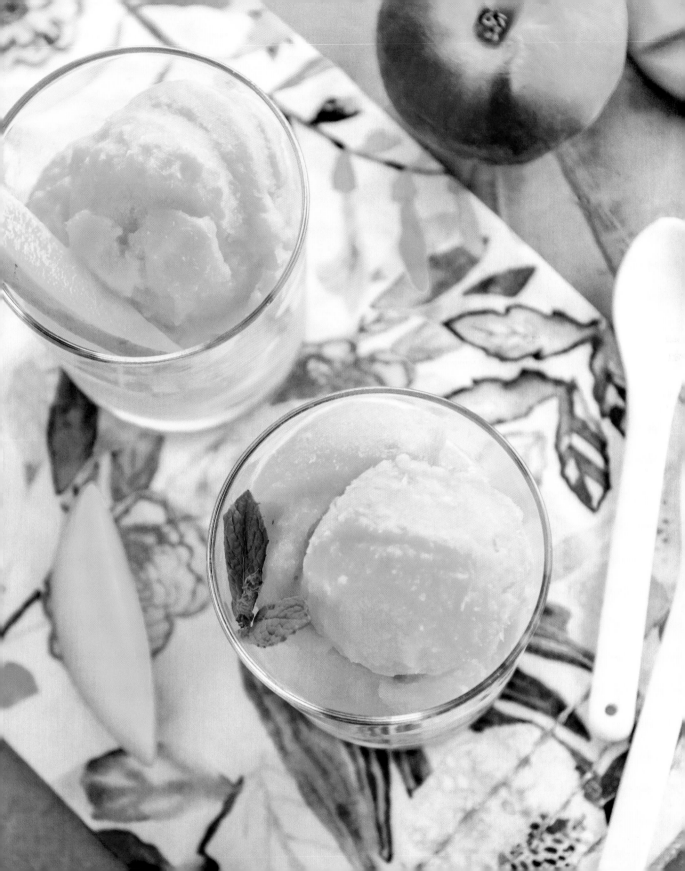

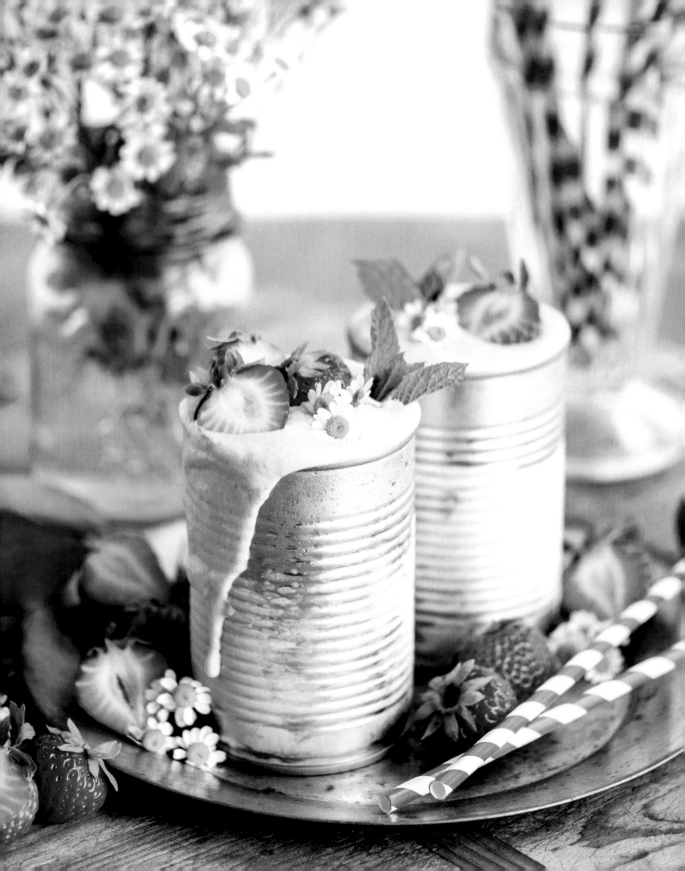

strawberry coconut shake

This simple plant-based alternative to a strawberry milkshake has passed the taste test with my kids and their friends—so trust me, it's a winner! Feel free to swap out the coconut milk for another nut milk you prefer. **SERVES 2**

1 can (13 ounces) full-fat coconut milk
1½ cups frozen strawberries

1 tablespoon pure maple syrup
1 teaspoon pure vanilla extract

In a blender, combine the coconut milk, strawberries, maple syrup, and vanilla and puree until smooth. Pour into 2 glasses and serve immediately, or transfer to an airtight container and keep refrigerated for several days or frozen for several weeks.

GLUTEN FREE, NUT FREE, VEGAN, DAIRY FREE

rawkstar tip

For an extra-thick shake, add to the blender ¼ cup presoaked raw cashews or 2 tablespoons cashew butter.

salted caramel bites

Oh, my goodness—these tasty little treats are loaded with sweetness, protein, and fiber. They will not only help with your sweet cravings but also nourish and satisfy your body. No empty calories here! Feel free to indulge! **MAKES 18 BITES**

1 cup raw cashews
1 cup soft and sticky Medjool dates,
    pitted

½ cup tahini
1 teaspoon pure vanilla extract
¼ teaspoon sea salt

1. In the bowl of a food processor fitted with the chopping blade, pulse the cashews until finely chopped. Add the dates and process until a thick, sticky paste forms. Stop to scrape down the sides of the bowl as needed.

2. Add the tahini, vanilla, and salt and process until the mixture forms a dough. If the mixture isn't sticking together well, add a tiny bit of water and process again.

3. Scoop out a heaping teaspoon of the mixture and roll into a ball about 1½ inches in diameter. Repeat to form approximately 18 balls. Freeze on a baking sheet until firm, then transfer to an airtight container and store at room temperature for up to 5 days.

GLUTEN FREE, VEGAN, DAIRY FREE

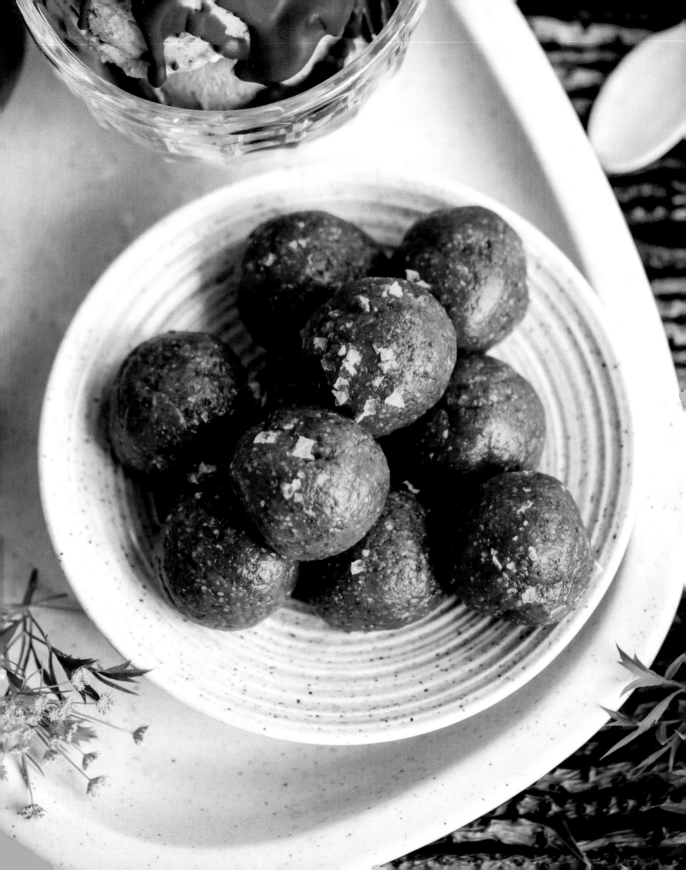

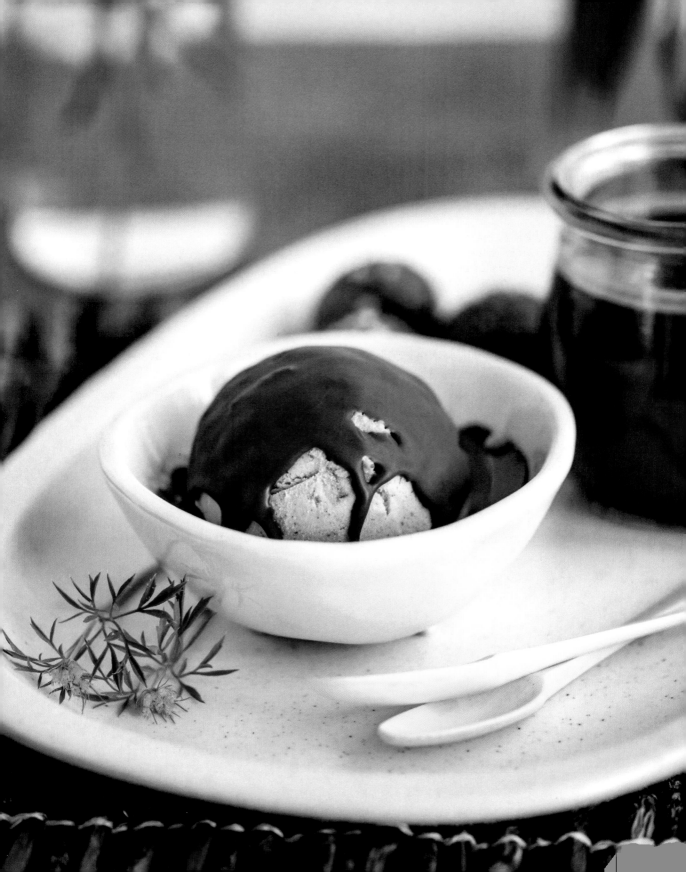

banana ice cream

When I got my first high-powered blender, I went crazy blending anything I could. Whole apples, hot soups, raw carrots, frozen bananas, and almonds were definitely part of the test. One of my favorite recipes from those early days was this ice cream that I created on a "Will it blend?" rampage. **SERVES 4**

4 ripe bananas, cut into 2-inch pieces
¼ cup almond butter
1 tablespoon pure vanilla extract
Pinch of ground cinnamon

Pinch of sea salt

SUGGESTED TOPPING
Chocolate Crackle (below)

1. Freeze the banana pieces for at least 4 hours.

2. In a high-powered blender, combine the bananas, almond butter, vanilla, cinnamon, and salt. Blend, stopping to push the bananas down and scrape down the sides. When the mixture is smooth and thick, like frozen yogurt, it's ready to eat. Or the mixture can be frozen until firm enough to scoop.

3. Serve in a bowl with the crackle sauce, if using. Store leftovers in an airtight container in the freezer for up to 2 weeks.

CHOCOLATE CRACKLE

Ryan and I spent the first few years of our marriage eating ice cream topped with Magic Shell. Once I read the ingredients label and saw what was in it, however, Magic Shell couldn't stay around. So I quickly found a DIY alternative to replace it. We've never wanted to go back! **SERVES 4**

1 bar (4 ounces) vegan dark chocolate, chopped

2 tablespoons organic virgin coconut oil
Pinch of sea salt

1. In a heatproof bowl set over a pan of simmering water, or in the top pan of a double boiler, melt the chocolate, oil, and sea salt. Stir until smooth.

2. Let cool slightly before drizzling over ice cream. Or transfer to a glass jar and refrigerate. To reheat the sauce, place the jar in a pan of hot water until the mixture has melted.

GLUTEN FREE, NUT FREE *(replace almond butter with coconut cream)*, VEGAN, DAIRY FREE

southern peach cobbler

When peach season comes to the South, things blow up . . . in a good way. We all start dreaming about what we're gonna make: peach tea, peach jam, peach smoothies, peach pancakes . . . it goes on and on. This simple peach cobbler is always on my list. **SERVES 12**

FOR FILLING
3 pounds peaches, peeled, pitted, and sliced (about 9 cups)
½ cup coconut sugar
2 tablespoons arrowroot powder
Juice of 1 lemon
1 teaspoon ground cinnamon
1 teaspoon pure vanilla extract
Pinch ground nutmeg

FOR TOPPING
1½ cups gluten-free all-purpose flour
½ cup fine stone-ground cornmeal
¼ cup coconut sugar

2 teaspoons baking powder
½ teaspoon baking soda
½ teaspoon sea salt
⅔ cup almond milk
2 teaspoons fresh lemon juice
1 large egg
1 teaspoon pure vanilla extract
½ cup extra-virgin coconut oil, chilled

FOR SERVING
Vanilla Bean Ice Cream (page 215)
Sliced almonds
Ground cinnamon

1. Preheat the oven to 400°F.

2. *To make the filling:* In a very large bowl, stir together the filling ingredients until well combined. Set aside.

3. *To make the topping:* In a medium bowl, whisk together the flour, cornmeal, coconut sugar, baking powder, baking soda, and sea salt. Set aside. Combine almond milk and lemon juice in a glass measuring cup and let stand for 2 to 3 minutes. Stir in the egg and vanilla until well combined. Add the chilled coconut oil to the dry ingredients. Working quickly, stir the oil into the dry ingredients with a fork until the mixture looks crumbly. Make a well in the center and add the liquid ingredients all at once. Quickly stir to just bring the dough together; don't overmix.

4. Transfer the peaches to a 9 x 13-inch baking dish or large cast-iron skillet. Drop mounds of the dough evenly over the peach filling. Bake, uncovered, for 45 minutes, or until the topping is golden and the filling is bubbling in the center. Let cool slightly before serving with ice cream and garnishing with almonds and cinnamon.

- -

DAIRY FREE, GLUTEN FREE

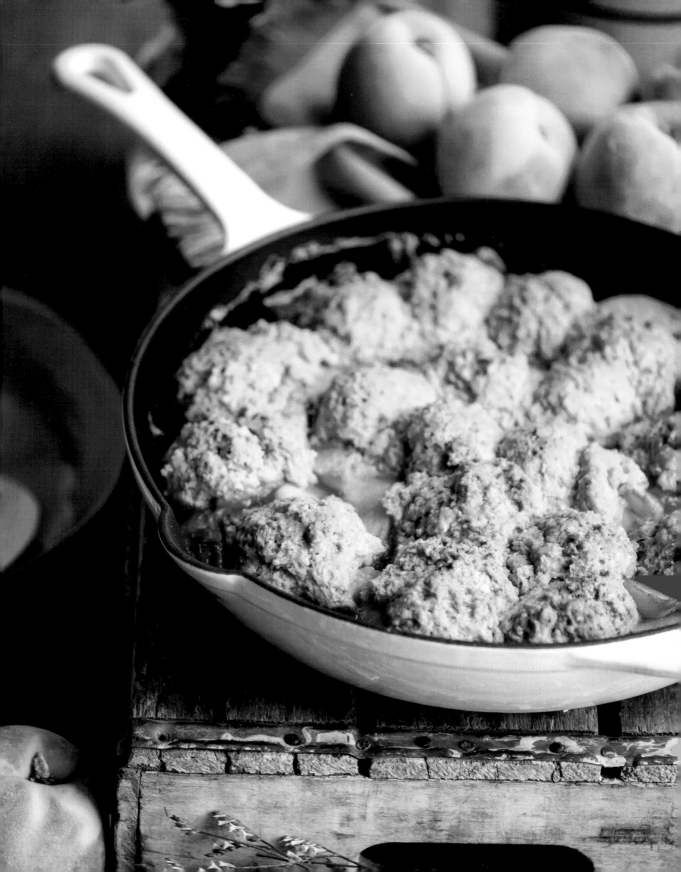

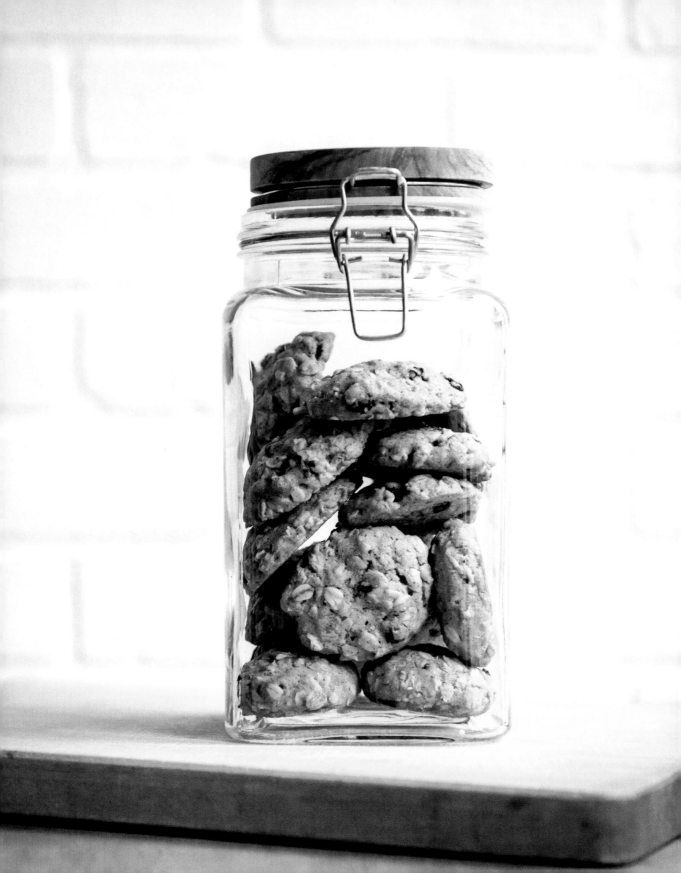

maple raisin cookies

The word *cookie* always makes me think "unhealthy," but these cookies are anything but. I guess you could think of them more like cookie-shaped granola bars. They are satisfying and delicious when dipped in a cup of almond milk. **MAKES 36 COOKIES**

1 cup whole wheat flour
1 teaspoon ground cinnamon
½ teaspoon baking powder
½ teaspoon baking soda
½ teaspoon sea salt
¼ teaspoon ground nutmeg
½ cup organic virgin coconut oil, at room temperature

⅓ cup almond butter
½ cup pure maple syrup
1 egg plus 1 egg yolk
1 teaspoon pure vanilla extract
1½ cups gluten-free rolled oats
¾ cup raisins

1. In a medium bowl, whisk together the flour, cinnamon, baking powder, baking soda, salt, and nutmeg.

2. In a stand mixer fitted with the paddle attachment, beat together the oil, almond butter, maple syrup, egg and egg yolk, and vanilla. Add the flour mixture, a little at a time, mixing after each addition until just combined. Stop to scrape down the sides as needed. Add the oats and raisins and mix again. Refrigerate the dough until firm.

3. Preheat the oven to 350°F. Line 2 baking sheets with parchment paper.

4. Using a mini ice cream scoop or a spoon, drop the dough onto the prepared baking sheets. Leave 2 inches between the cookies. Using your palm or the bottom of a drinking glass, press down on the cookies to flatten. Bake for about 10 minutes for softer cookies, about 12 minutes for crisper cookies.

5. Let the cookies cool slightly on the baking sheets before transferring to racks. Cool completely, then store in an airtight container. These will keep fresh for about a week at room temperature, or they can be frozen for several months.

- -

GLUTEN FREE *(replace flour with ¾ cup gluten-free all-purpose flour)*, NUT FREE *(replace almond butter with sunflower butter)*, VEGAN *(replace egg and yolk with 1 banana)*, DAIRY FREE

thin mint cookies

I can't remember what I had for dinner last week, but I can still recite the Girl Scout pledge. It's ingrained deep in my brain. When we Scouts would go door to door selling cookies, Thin Mints were always the top seller. People would buy a bunch to store in the freezer and enjoy all year long. When I started caring about the ingredients I was putting in my body, Thin Mints had to go—until I decided it was time to create a healthier alternative that you can make any time you want. **MAKES 48 COOKIES**

FOR COOKIES
1 cup almond flour
½ cup arrowroot powder
½ cup cacao powder
1 teaspoon baking powder
¼ teaspoon sea salt
½ cup organic virgin coconut oil, at room temperature
½ cup coconut sugar
1 egg
½ teaspoon pure peppermint extract

FOR CHOCOLATE COATING
1 bag (12 ounces) vegan semisweet chocolate chips
2 teaspoons organic virgin coconut oil
¼ teaspoon pure peppermint extract

1. *To make the cookies:* In a medium bowl, whisk together the almond flour, arrowroot powder, cacao powder, baking powder, and salt.

2. In a large mixing bowl, and using a hand mixer, beat together the oil, sugar, egg, and peppermint extract. Add the flour mixture and beat until well combined.

3. Place a piece of parchment paper, waxed paper, or plastic wrap on a clean, flat surface. Turn out the dough onto the paper or wrap and form into a log that is 12 inches long and about 2 inches in diameter. Wrap tightly and refrigerate or freeze until firm enough to slice.

4. Preheat the oven to 350°F. Line 2 baking sheets with parchment paper.

5. Unwrap the dough. Using a very sharp, thin knife, cut the dough into 48 rounds that are ¼ inch thick. (If the dough has been frozen, let it warm up a bit for easier slicing.) Place the rounds on the prepared baking sheets, leaving a little space between each to accommodate any spreading. Bake for 8 minutes, or until the edges and centers are set. For crisper cookies, bake longer.

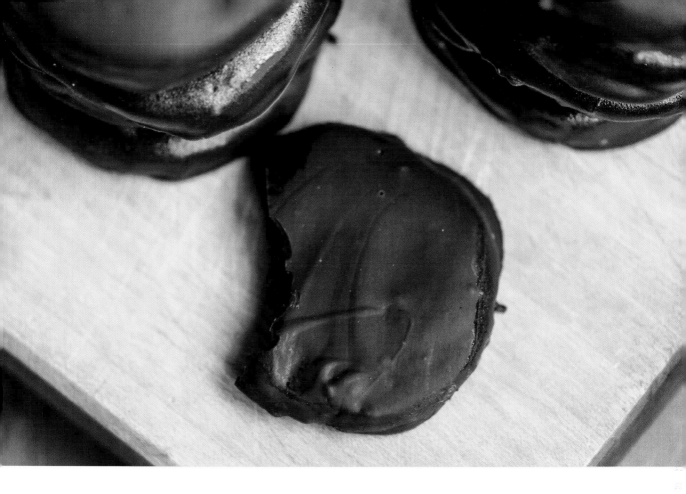

6. Let cool completely on the baking sheets. (Keep the parchment paper–lined baking sheets handy for dipping the cookies.)

7. *To make the chocolate coating:* In a heatproof glass bowl set over a pan of simmering water, melt the chocolate chips, oil, and peppermint extract.

8. Working with 1 cookie at a time, put the cookie on a fork and lower it into the melted chocolate until completely coated. Tap gently so excess chocolate falls back into the bowl. Drag the bottom of the fork over the edge of the bowl to remove any extra chocolate. Place the cookies on the lined baking sheets. Allow the chocolate to set up (refrigerating or freezing will speed the process), then store the cookies in an airtight container between layers of parchment or waxed paper to prevent them from sticking together. The thin mints keep best in a cool, dry place or in the freezer.

GLUTEN FREE, NUT FREE *(replace the almond flour with gluten-free all-purpose flour),* VEGAN *(replace egg with 1 "chia egg": mix 1 tablespoon chia seeds with 3 tablespoons water; let sit for 10 minutes before adding to recipe),* DAIRY FREE

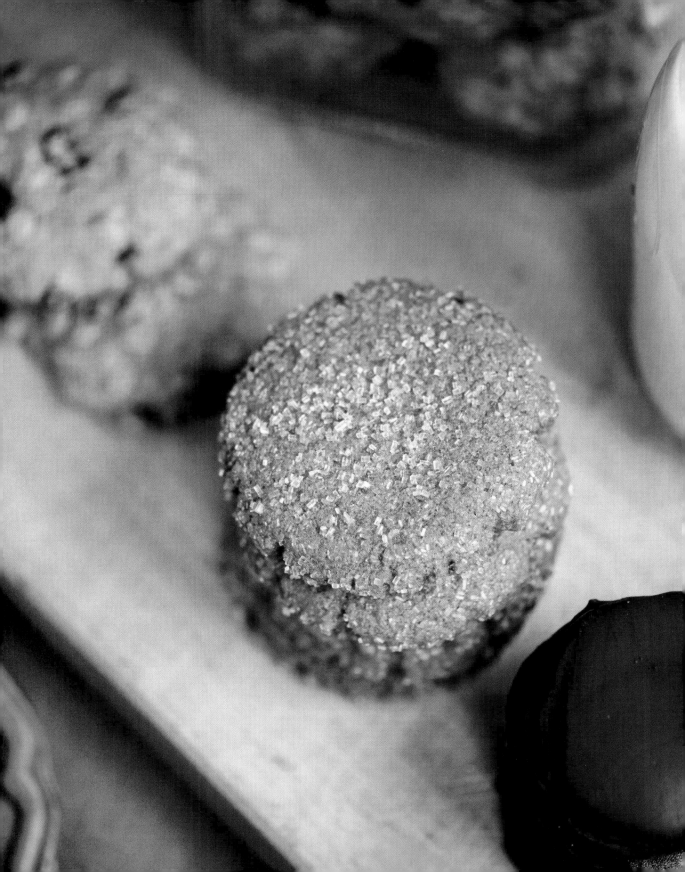

honey-ginger cookies

It's amazing how much our parents' food choices can shape our own. My mom passed down her love of Neccos and coffee. My dad passed down his love for black licorice and, of course, ginger cookies. The only difference is he prefers the rock-hard cookies—aka "hockey pucks" to us as kids—and I prefer the soft and chewy ones. Since this is my recipe book, I made them the way I like. **MAKES 3 DOZEN COOKIES**

1½ cups white whole wheat flour
2 tablespoons ground flaxseed
1½ teaspoons ground ginger
½ teaspoon ground cinnamon
Pinch of ground cloves
1 teaspoon baking soda
½ teaspoon sea salt

½ cup organic virgin coconut oil, melted
½ cup honey
¼ cup blackstrap molasses
1 egg
1 teaspoon finely grated fresh ginger
½ cup organic sugar for rolling (optional)

1. In a medium bowl, whisk together the flour, flaxseed, ground ginger, cinnamon, cloves, baking soda, and salt.

2. In a large mixing bowl, and using an electric mixer on medium-high speed, beat the oil, honey, molasses, egg, and fresh ginger until well combined. With the mixer on low speed, add half of the flour mixture and beat until just combined. Add the remaining flour mixture and beat again. The dough will be fairly sticky.

3. Cover the bowl and refrigerate for at least 1 hour and up to 5 hours, or until the dough holds its shape when rolled into a ball.

4. Preheat the oven to 350°F. Line 2 baking sheets with parchment paper.

5. Roll pieces of dough into 1-inch balls. Roll the balls in the sugar, if using. Place 2 inches apart on the prepared baking sheets. Using your palm or the bottom of a drinking glass, press down on the cookies to flatten.

6. Bake for 8 minutes. Let cool completely on the pan; hot cookies will be too tender to pick up. They will set up as they cool. Transfer to an airtight container and store in a cool, dry place or freeze.

GLUTEN FREE, DAIRY FREE

lemon–poppy seed cake

I grew up in the Antelope Valley, a suburb outside of Los Angeles, and our claim to fame is the bright orange poppy fields that bloom in the spring. People travel from all over the world to experience the fiery orange natural beauty. It's truly breathtaking. This recipe is in honor of my hometown. I hope you have a recipe that does that for you, but if not, we can share this one! **SERVES 8**

½ cup organic virgin coconut oil, plus more for greasing pan
2 cups all-purpose flour
1 teaspoon baking powder
½ teaspoon baking soda
½ teaspoon sea salt
4 eggs
¾ cup pure maple syrup
¾ cup canned full-fat coconut milk

6 tablespoons fresh lemon juice
1 tablespoon finely grated lemon peel
2 teaspoons pure vanilla extract
½ teaspoon lemon extract
½ teaspoon pure almond extract
4 tablespoons poppy seeds

FOR SERVING
Vanilla Bean Ice Cream (page 215)
Fresh berries

1. Preheat the oven to 350°F. Generously grease a loaf pan with oil.

2. In a medium bowl, whisk together the flour, baking powder, baking soda, and salt.

3. In a large mixing bowl, whisk together the ½ cup coconut oil, eggs, maple syrup, coconut milk, lemon juice, lemon peel, vanilla, lemon extract, and almond extract. Add the flour mixture and whisk until smooth. Fold in the poppy seeds.

4. Pour the batter into the prepared pan. Bake for 50 minutes, or until the loaf is golden and springs back on top when lightly pressed and a wooden pick inserted in the center comes out clean. Let cool for 10 minutes in the pan, then turn out onto a rack.

5. Let cool completely before serving. Slice and serve topped with vegan ice cream and fresh berries.

GLUTEN FREE *(replace flour with gluten-free all-purpose flour)*, NUT FREE, VEGAN *(swap the eggs for 1 cup applesauce)*, DAIRY FREE

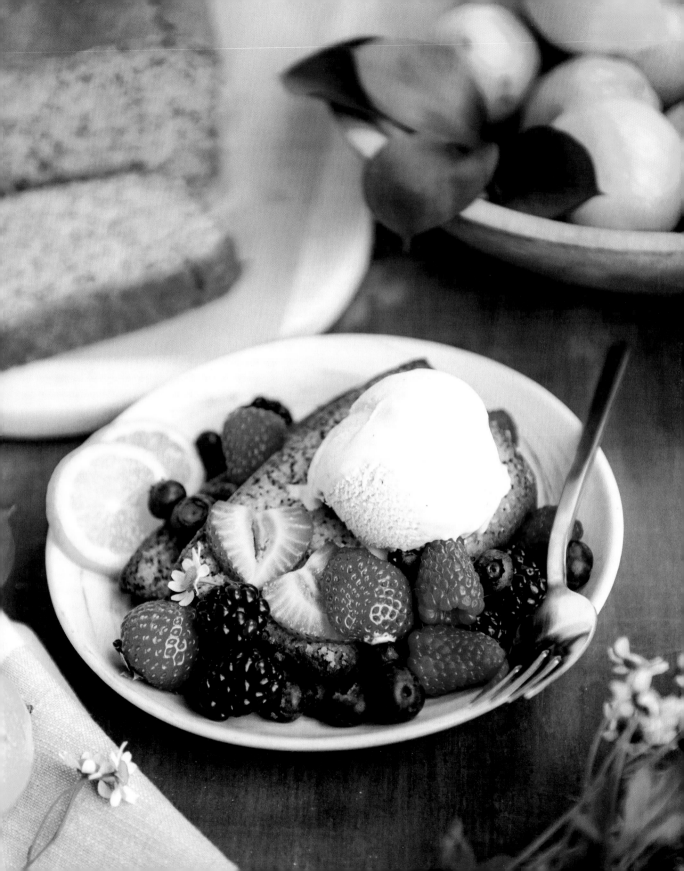

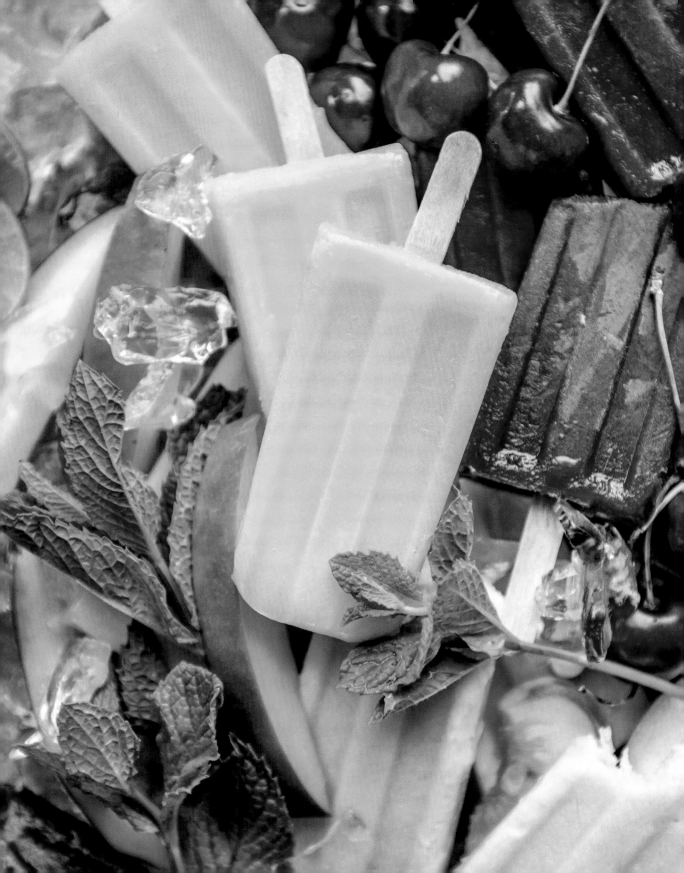

fresh fruit pops

Since I don't have a swimming pool, we use ice pops to cool off in the hot, humid dog days of summer. This trio has a little something for everyone—Jackson loves the mango ones; Clare is all about the cherry lime; and I'm obsessed with the peaches and cream. Make a bunch ahead and store in the freezer for a simple, all-natural refresher. The ice-pop mold used for testing contained 6 molds with a ¾-cup capacity each. **MAKES 6 POPS**

MANGO MOJITO

4 mangoes, pitted and peeled
   (about 3 cups cubed)
⅓ cup organic cane sugar
¾ cup water
5 mint leaves
¼ cup fresh lime juice

PEACHES 'N' CREAM

3 cups peaches, sliced
⅓ cup organic cane sugar
1 cup full-fat coconut milk
1 tablespoon fresh lemon juice
1 teaspoon pure vanilla extract
½ teaspoon almond extract

CHERRY LIME

3 cups fresh or frozen cherries, pitted
⅓ cup organic cane sugar
¾ cup water
¼ cup fresh lime juice

1. Choose the flavor you want to make. Place the fruit, sugar, liquid, and any other ingredients into a blender. Puree until smooth. Tap the blender jar (with the lid on) against the counter to help remove excess air bubbles.

2. Pour the mixture into the ice pop molds and freeze until firm, 4 hours or preferably overnight.

- -

GLUTEN FREE, NUT FREE, VEGAN, DAIRY FREE

tri-protein chocolate squares

Chickpeas, almond butter, and rolled oats have combined forces (unexpectedly!) to create this sweet and nutty treat that's packed with healthy fats and protein. **MAKES 16 SQUARES**

FOR BLONDIE LAYER
1 can (15 ounces) chickpeas, drained and rinsed
⅓ cup pure maple syrup
½ cup almond butter
2 teaspoons pure vanilla extract
1 teaspoon baking powder
½ teaspoon baking soda
½ teaspoon sea salt
¼ teaspoon ground cinnamon
½ cup gluten-free rolled oats

FOR ALMOND BUTTER LAYER
½ cup almond butter
1 tablespoon pure maple syrup
1 tablespoon organic virgin coconut oil, melted
Pinch of sea salt

FOR CHOCOLATE TOPPING
4 ounces vegan dark chocolate, chopped
2 tablespoons unsweetened plain almond milk

1. Preheat the oven to 350°F. Grease a 9 × 9-inch baking dish.

2. *To make the blondie layer:* In a food processor, combine the chickpeas and maple syrup and process until thick and creamy. Add the almond butter, vanilla, baking powder, baking soda, salt, and cinnamon. Process until smooth. Add the oats and pulse a few times until they are a little broken up. Transfer to the prepared dish.

3. Bake for 20 minutes, or until the center is set. They will still look a little wet in the center and will continue to set up as they cool. Let cool completely.

4. *To make the almond butter layer:* In a medium bowl, whisk together the almond butter, maple syrup, oil, and salt until smooth. Pour over the cooled bars and spread in an even layer. Chill for 30 minutes, or until set.

5. *To make the chocolate topping:* In a heatproof glass bowl set over a pan of simmering water, melt the chocolate and almond milk. Stir well. Let cool slightly, then pour over the almond butter layer and spread evenly to the pan edges.

6. Chill until firm enough to cut into bars. Store in the refrigerator for up to 1 week.

GLUTEN FREE, NUT FREE *(replace almond milk with coconut milk; replace almond butter with sunflower butter)*, VEGAN, DAIRY FREE

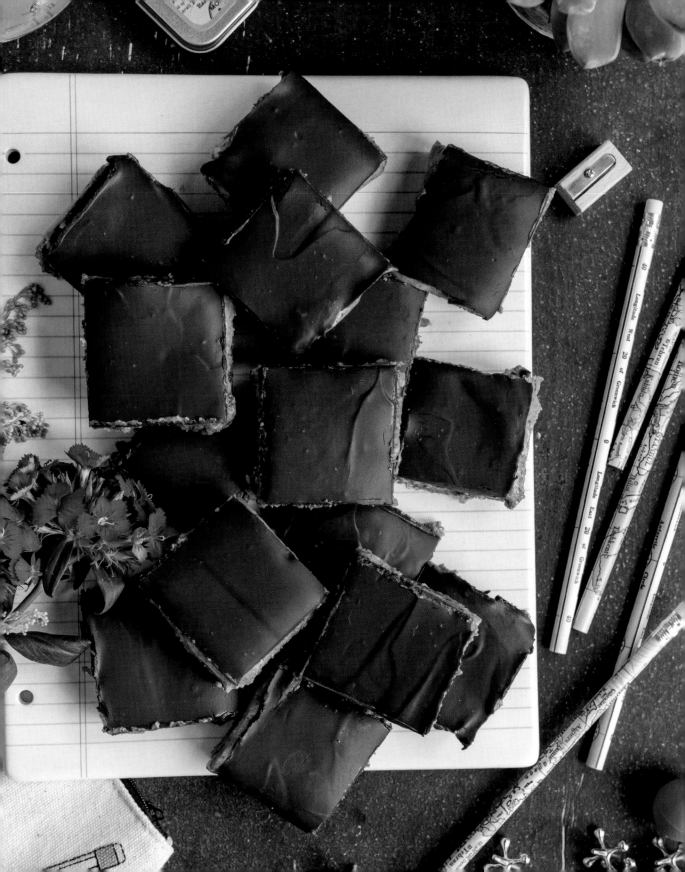

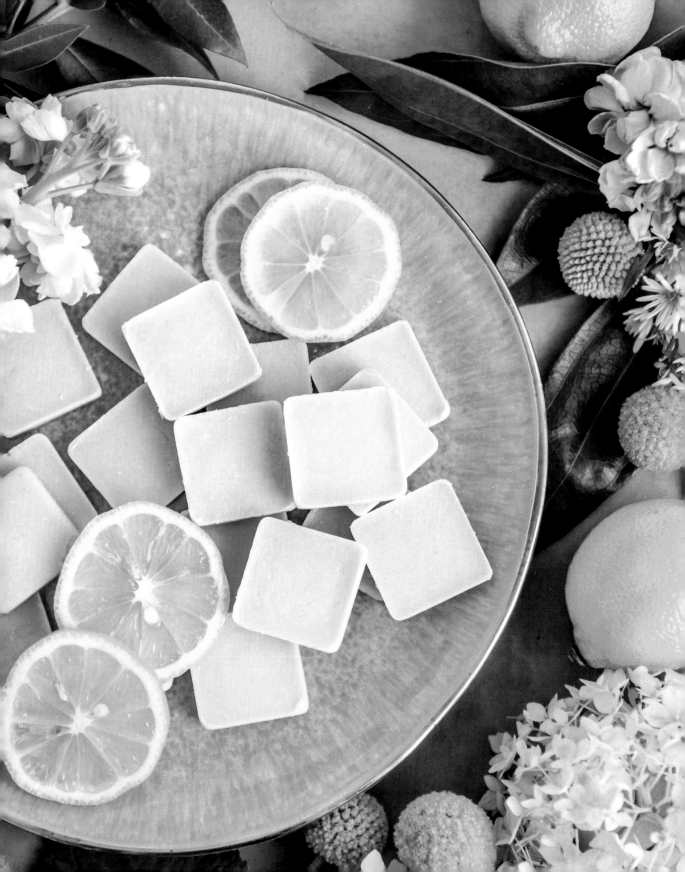

lemon tart meltaways

Getting enough healthy fat on a daily basis takes a bit of work, yet the results are worth it. Improved digestion, supple skin, and blazing energy all encourage me to pack in the healthy fats as I get, well, older. These lemon meltaways are essentially healthy "fat bombs," which make a great quick afternoon snack. I should warn you—you really have to like lemons to like these tart treats. **MAKES 3 DOZEN MELTAWAYS**

½ cup raw cashews
2 tablespoons pure maple syrup
2 tablespoons fresh lemon juice, plus more to taste

½ cup organic virgin coconut oil
Pinch of sea salt

1. Place a baking sheet lined with waxed paper in the freezer.

2. In a blender or food processor, blend or process the cashews until finely ground. Add the maple syrup and lemon juice and pulse a few times. Add the oil and salt and puree until smooth and creamy.

3. Remove the cold baking sheet from the freezer and drop ½ tablespoonfuls of the cashew mixture onto it. Return the pan to the freezer. (Depending on the size of the baking sheet, you may have to make the meltaways in batches.) When the drops are solid, peel them from the waxed paper and store in the freezer in an airtight freezer container.

GLUTEN FREE, VEGAN, DAIRY FREE

vanilla cupcakes

I made these cupcakes for a get-together with my family in Boise, and everyone—including my cousin Gabe—loved them and had no clue something was missing . . . like eggs and milk! That's when I decided it was time to put this recipe in a book so others can enjoy them, too.

MAKES 12 CUPCAKES

1½ cups unbleached all-purpose flour
1 teaspoon baking powder
½ teaspoon sea salt
¾ cup pure maple syrup, at room temperature
½ cup organic virgin coconut oil, at room temperature

1 teaspoon pure vanilla extract
¾ cup unsweetened plain almond milk, at room temperature

FOR SERVING
Ryan's Fudge Frosting (page 243) or Jen's Strawberry Frosting (page 243)

1. Preheat the oven to 350°F. Line a standard 12-cup muffin pan with paper liners.

2. In a medium bowl, whisk together the flour, baking powder, and salt.

3. In the bowl of a stand mixer fitted with the paddle attachment, or in a large bowl and using a whisk, beat the maple syrup and oil for about 3 minutes, or until creamy. Beat in the vanilla.

4. Starting and ending with the dry ingredients, add one-third of the flour mixture to the maple mixture alternately with the almond milk. Beat only until combined. Stop to scrape down the sides of the bowl as needed.

5. Divide the batter evenly among the paper-lined cups in the prepared muffin pan. Bake for 15 to 20 minutes, checking after 15 minutes, until the cupcakes are lightly golden and springy to the touch.

6. Let the cupcakes cool for a few minutes in the pan, then remove to a rack to finish cooling. Frost and serve.

- -

GLUTEN FREE *(replace flour with gluten-free all-purpose flour)*, VEGAN, DAIRY FREE

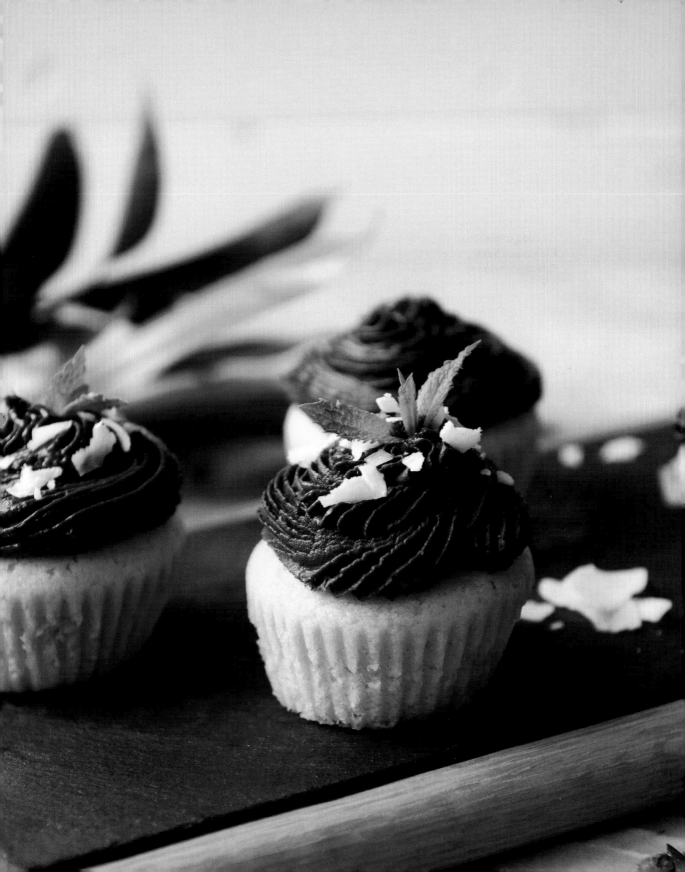

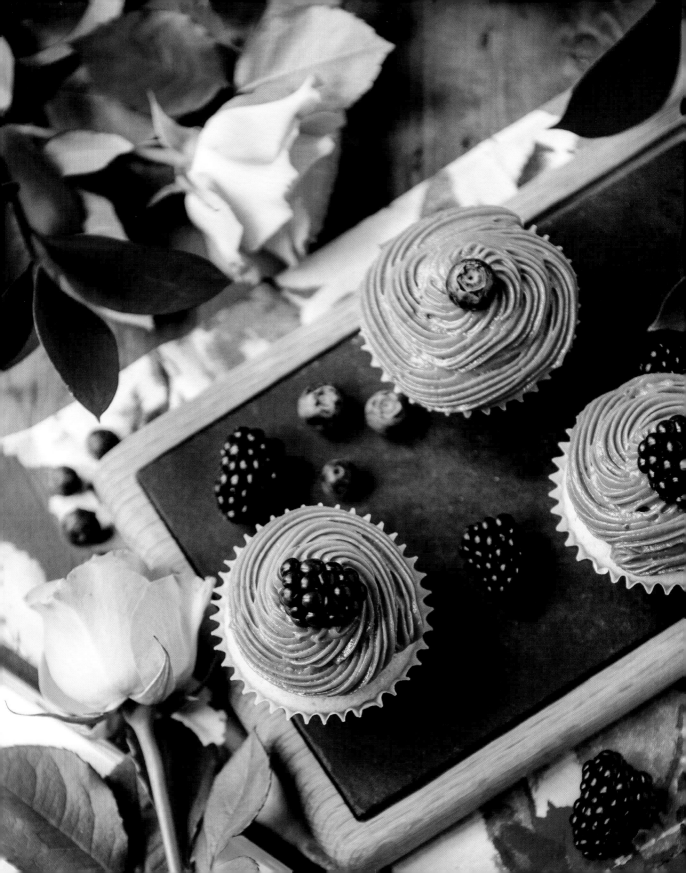

ryan's fudge frosting

My husband, Ryan, is the chocolate lover in our family. He appreciates when we include chocolate for dessert, which isn't that often since I'm a fruit kinda gal and do all of the baking. This one is for him and all the other chocolate lovers out there—enjoy! **MAKES 2 CUPS**

1½ cups vegan semisweet chocolate chips
¼ cup unsweetened plain almond milk
¼ cup organic virgin coconut oil

1 teaspoon pure vanilla extract
Pinch of sea salt
2 tablespoons honey

Combine the ingredients in a saucepan over medium-low heat. Stir until the chocolate melts. Transfer to a mixing bowl and refrigerate until cold and firm to the touch. Using an electric hand mixer, beat on medium speed for 3 minutes, or until thick and fudgy. Add a little extra coconut oil if frosting seems too dry.

GLUTEN FREE, NUT FREE *(replace almond milk with coconut milk)*, VEGAN *(replace honey with brown rice syrup)*, DAIRY FREE

jen's strawberry frosting

Hands down, this is the best-tasting vegan frosting I have ever had, and I will make it again and again—and eat it all without remorse! The secret is using freeze-dried strawberries, which have had the moisture removed and help the frosting stay thick. **MAKES 2 CUPS**

1½ cups raw cashews
3 tablespoons fresh lemon juice, divided
½ cup organic virgin coconut oil, melted
½ cup pure maple syrup

2 cups freeze-dried strawberries
1 teaspoon pure vanilla extract
Pinch of sea salt
1 teaspoon freeze-dried beet powder (optional, for extra color)

Soak the cashews for 2 hours in the lemon juice and enough water to cover. Drain and rinse well. In a blender, puree the cashews and the remaining ingredients until smooth. Refrigerate until the frosting firms up enough to spread.

GLUTEN FREE, VEGAN, DAIRY FREE

cacao mug cake

This dessert could not be easier to make—mix up the ingredients in a mug, pop in the oven, and dig into chocolatey heaven. If you're feeling in the mood for something extra decadent, add a tablespoon or two of vegan dark chocolate chips on top of the batter before baking. Or serve with a small scoop of Vanilla Bean Ice Cream (page 215). **SERVES 1**

1 egg
2 tablespoons pure maple syrup
¼ cup almond flour
2 tablespoons cacao powder, plus more for sprinkling

1 tablespoon organic virgin coconut oil, melted
1 tablespoon unsweetened plain almond milk
1 teaspoon pure vanilla extract
Pinch of sea salt

1. Preheat the oven to 350°F.

2. Crack the egg into an ovenproof mug or other container. Beat with a fork. Add the maple syrup and beat again. Then add the almond flour, cacao powder, oil, almond milk, vanilla, and salt and stir until well combined.

3. Bake for 15 minutes for a fudgy cake or 20 minutes for a cakey texture. Test with a wooden pick to make sure it's cooked through. *Note:* The cake will rise up a bit during baking and sink as it cools.

4. Serve warm with a sprinkling of cacao powder.

GLUTEN FREE *(replace flour with gluten-free oat flour)*, NUT FREE *(replace almond milk with coconut milk)*, VEGAN *(replace the egg with 1 tablespoon flaxseed plus 3 tablespoons water)*, DAIRY FREE

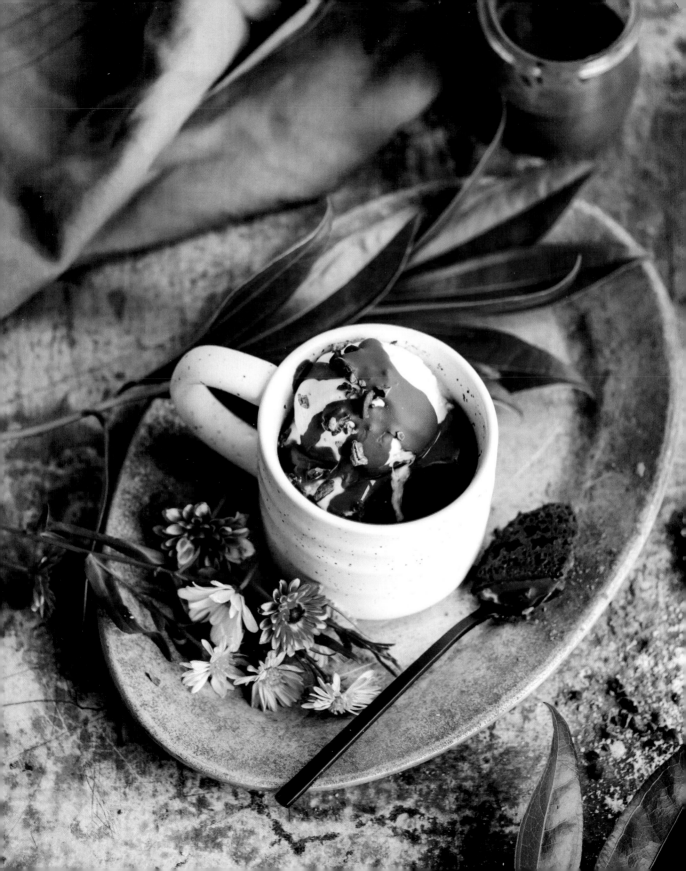

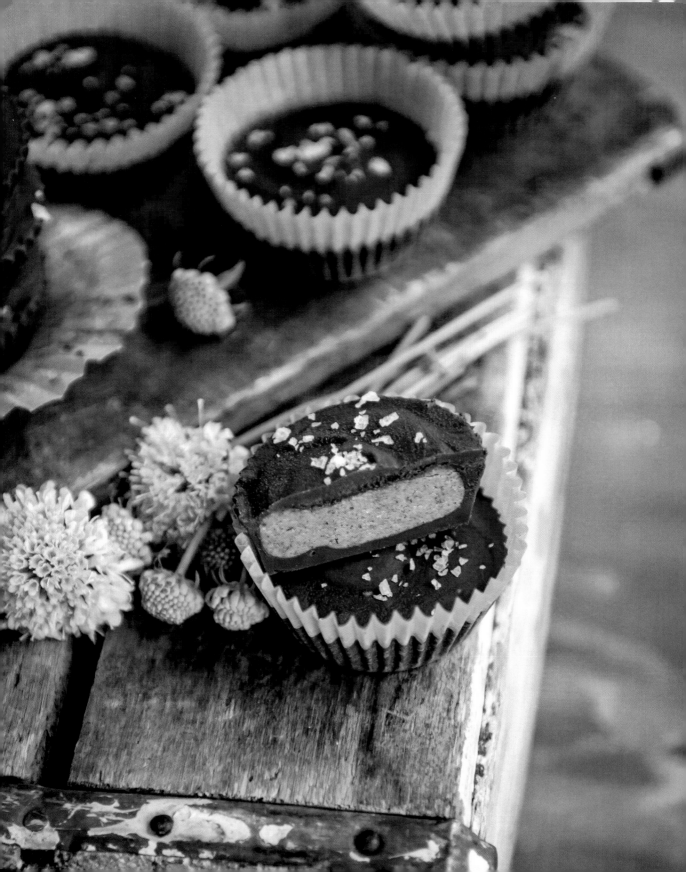

almond butter cups

I've never been one to get excited about a chocolate treat, until I made these gems. They have the perfect combination of chocolate, coconut oil, and almond butter—it's hard to stop at one. I recommend freezing the rest so it's more difficult to get to them if you, too, have trouble saying no to a good thing. **MAKES 12 CUPS**

FOR FILLING
¾ cup almond butter
1 tablespoon pure maple syrup
Pinch of sea salt

FOR CHOCOLATE COATING
2 teaspoons organic virgin coconut oil
2 cups vegan semisweet chocolate, chopped

1. Line a standard 12-cup muffin pan with paper liners.

2. *To make the filling:* In a medium bowl, stir together the almond butter, maple syrup, and salt.

3. *To make the chocolate coating:* In a heatproof glass bowl set over a pan of simmering water, melt the chocolate and oil. (Alternatively, place the chocolate and oil in a microwaveable bowl and microwave at 50% power in 30- to 60-second intervals, stirring between each interval. Be careful not to let the chocolate get too hot or it will burn.) When almost all of the chocolate has melted, remove from the heat or microwave. Stir gently until the chocolate is smooth, being careful not to create air bubbles.

4. Spoon a tablespoonful of melted chocolate into each paper-lined cup. Use the tip of the spoon to push some of the chocolate up the sides of the liner, but make sure enough remains to coat the bottom.

5. Spoon 1 tablespoon of the almond butter mixture into each cup. Gently press down if the mixture is thick instead of runny.

6. Immediately spoon a scant tablespoon of melted chocolate over the almond butter. Use the back of the spoon to make sure the chocolate covers the whole patty and drips down the sides to the chocolate on the bottom. This will seal the almond filling inside.

7. Place the muffin pan in the fridge for 45 to 60 minutes, or until the cups set up completely before serving. Store in an airtight container. These are best stored in the fridge, and they can also be frozen for several months.

GLUTEN FREE, NUT FREE *(replace almond butter with sunflower butter)*, VEGAN, DAIRY FREE

baked apple crisp in a jar

It's no secret—I love mason jars for green smoothies! But I also love them for other things, like making individual desserts. Does it get any more adorable than this?! The sweet crisp topping is pretty irresistible. I recommend serving these warm with a scoop of Vanilla Bean Ice Cream (page 215). **SERVES 4**

FOR FILLING
4 green apples, peeled or unpeeled, cored, and diced
1 teaspoon ground cinnamon
½ teaspoon ground nutmeg
Pinch of sea salt
¼ cup pure maple syrup
2 tablespoons fresh lemon juice

FOR TOPPING
1 cup gluten-free rolled oats
½ cup whole wheat flour
½ cup chopped pecans
¼ cup organic virgin coconut oil, melted, plus more for greasing jars
¼ cup pure maple syrup
½ teaspoon sea salt

1. Preheat the oven to 350°F. Grease the insides of 4 pint-size mason jars.

2. *To make the filling:* In a large bowl, stir together the apples, cinnamon, nutmeg, salt, maple syrup, and lemon juice. Divide the mixture evenly between the jars. Tap the jars gently on the counter to help the apples settle into the bottom.

3. *To make the topping:* In another medium bowl, stir together the oats, flour, pecans, oil, maple syrup, and salt. Spoon 2 tablespoons of the mixture into each jar. Place the jars on a baking sheet, cover with foil, and bake for 25 minutes. Remove the foil and bake for 3 to 5 minutes, or until the top is crisp. Serve warm or at room temperature.

GLUTEN FREE *(replace flour with gluten-free all-purpose flour)*, NUT FREE *(remove pecans)*, VEGAN, DAIRY FREE

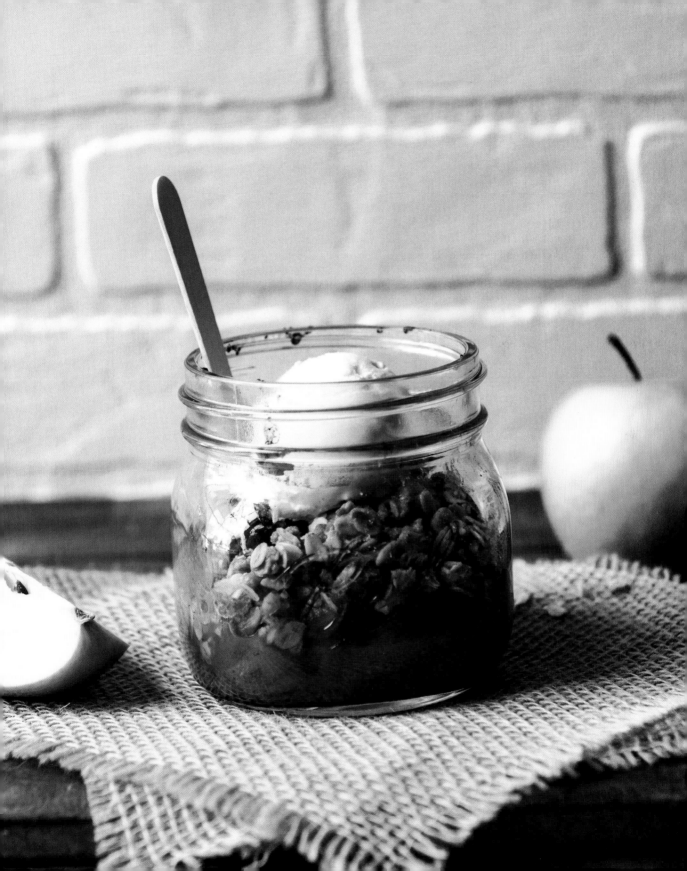

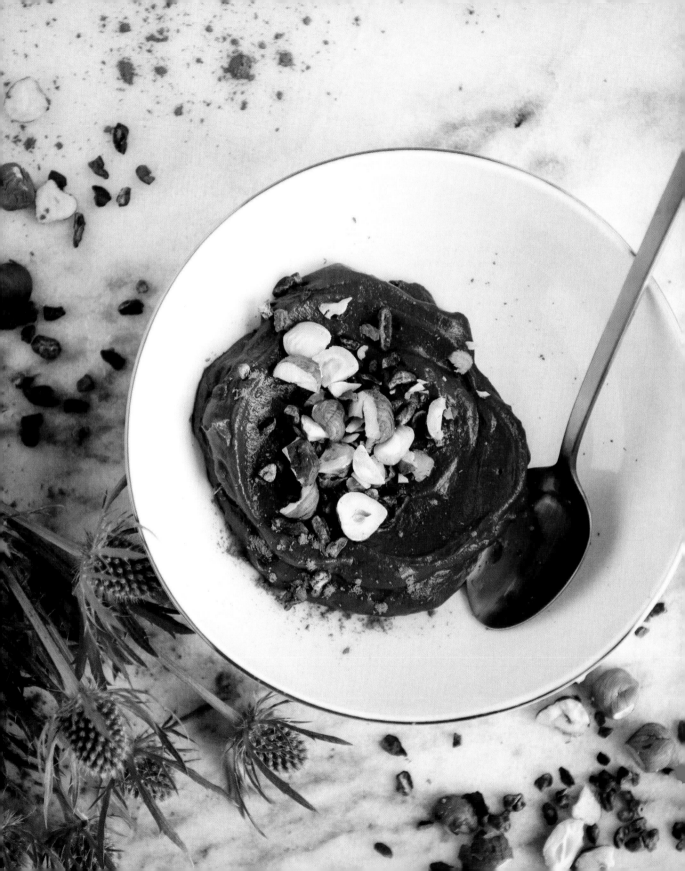

cacao pudding

At first glance, you may think the ingredients sound like a strange combo . . . and don't avocados exist solely for guacamole anyway? Nope! Avocados are actually a fruit chock-full of healthy fats, and they just so happen to make one heck of a creamy pudding. With this pudding's antioxidant-rich cacao, you'll be addicted after the first bite. **SERVES 2**

1 ripe avocado, halved and pitted
2 tablespoons cacao powder
1 tablespoon pure maple syrup

1 teaspoon pure vanilla extract
Pinch of sea salt
2 tablespoons hazelnuts, chopped

1. In a blender or food processor, combine the avocado, cacao powder, maple syrup, vanilla, and salt. Puree until smooth. The mixture will be really thick. Stop to scrape down the sides as needed.

2. Transfer to 2 bowls, cover, and chill until ready to serve. Sprinkle each bowl with 1 tablespoon hazelnuts.

GLUTEN FREE, NUT FREE *(remove hazelnuts)*, VEGAN, DAIRY FREE

cherry chocolate bark

I love it when I can make a recipe that is as insanely decadent as it is insanely healthy. This bark is right up there, thanks to its protein-rich almonds, antioxidant-packed cherries, and flavonoid-rich bittersweet chocolate. Chocolate lovers, enjoy this gem. **SERVES 8**

1 cup vegan semisweet chocolate chips
1 cup sliced almonds

1 cup dried tart cherries, chopped
½ teaspoon flaky sea salt, for sprinkling

1. Line a rimmed baking sheet with parchment paper and place in the fridge or freezer to get very cold.

2. In a heatproof glass bowl set over a pan of simmering water, melt the chocolate, stirring occasionally. Be careful not to let water droplets get into the bowl or the chocolate will seize.

3. Remove the bowl from the heat (or the microwave) when some pieces of unmelted chocolate still remain. Stir well until the remaining chocolate melts, but do not stir too vigorously or air bubbles will form.

4. Pour the melted chocolate onto the chilled prepared pan and use a thin spatula to spread it evenly almost to the edges of the pan. Immediately sprinkle the almonds and cherries evenly over the chocolate, followed by a sprinkling of salt. Refrigerate until firm.

5. Break the bark into pieces and store in an airtight container in the refrigerator for up to 1 week.

GLUTEN FREE, VEGAN, DAIRY FREE

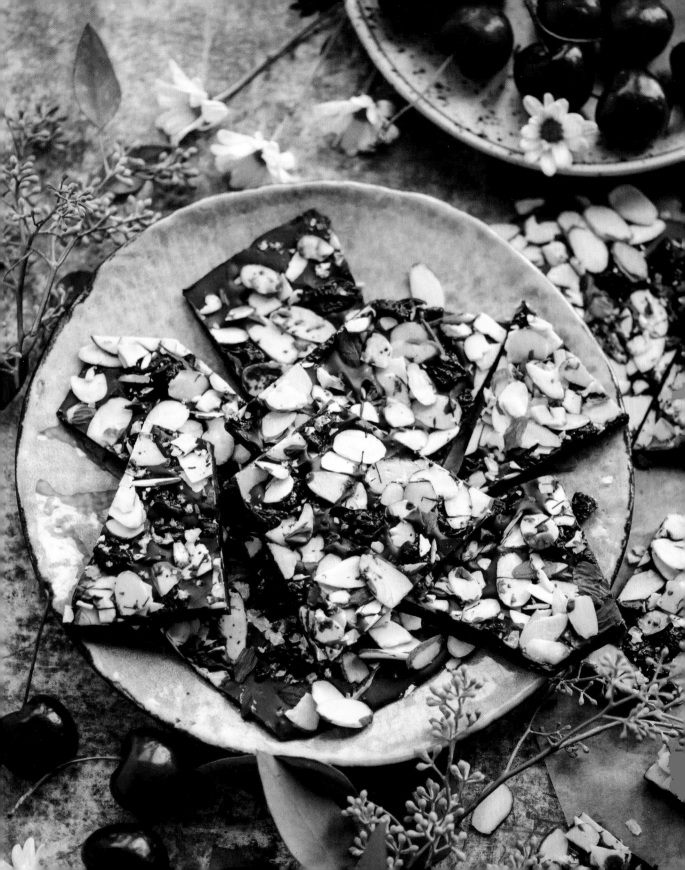

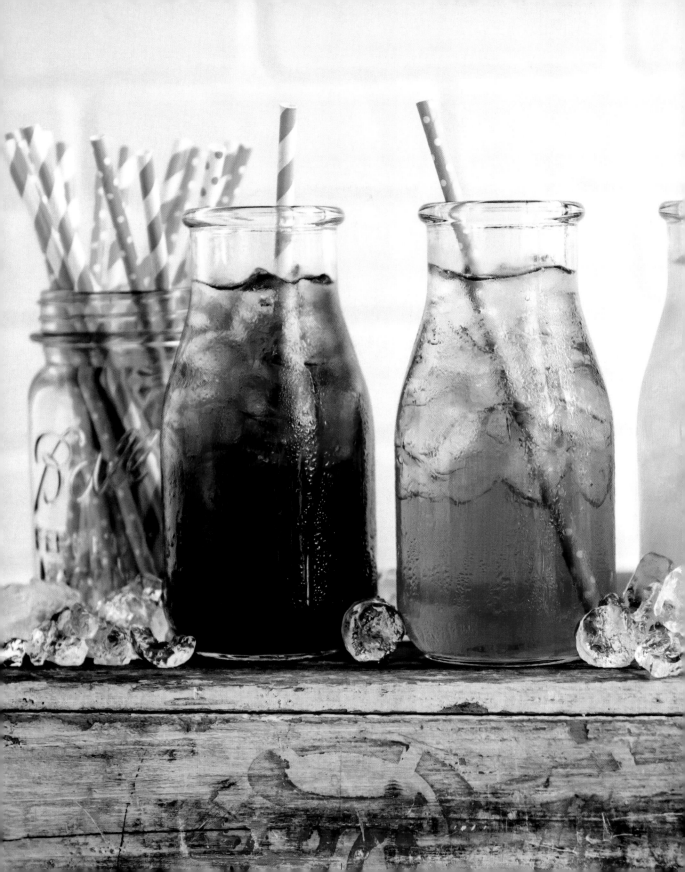

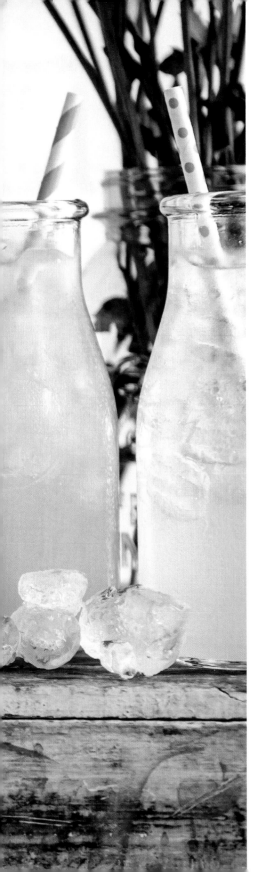

beverages

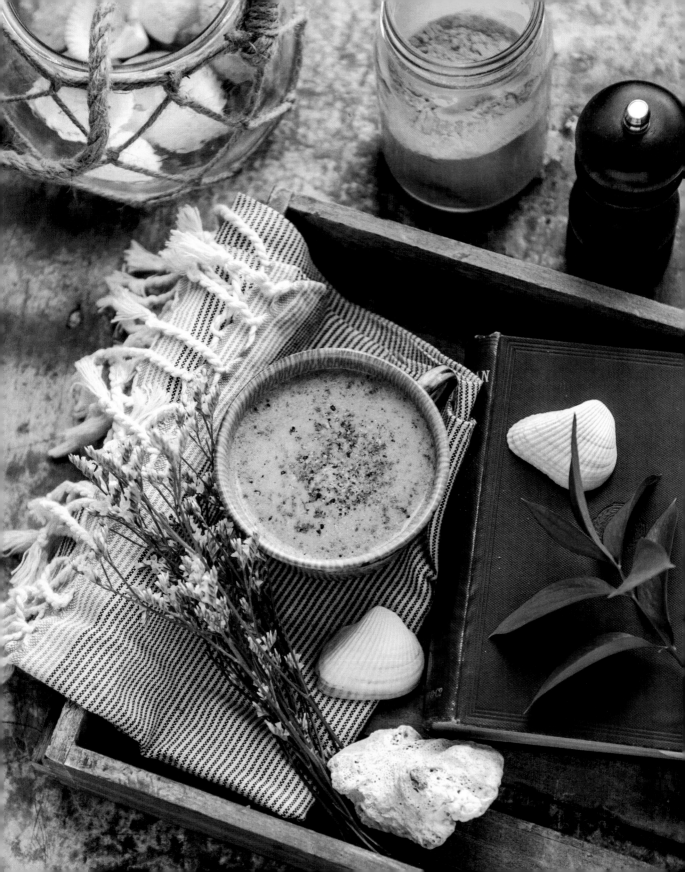

golden turmeric milk

Turmeric and ginger are superheros when it comes to fighting inflammation. They are also really good for warming up your insides on a cold night, which is when you'll find me sipping on this drink. I know the black pepper may seem strange, but it's essential for the efficacy of the turmeric. If the turmeric flavor is too strong for you, feel free to start with less and work up to as much as you can tolerate. **SERVES 1**

½ teaspoon ground turmeric
¼ teaspoon ground cinnamon
Pinch of ground black pepper
½ teaspoon grated fresh ginger

1 cup canned full-fat coconut milk
1 teaspoon raw honey
1 tablespoon organic virgin coconut oil

1. In a small saucepan, combine the turmeric, cinnamon, pepper, and ginger. Whisk in the coconut milk, honey, and oil. Heat over medium heat for 5 minutes, until very hot but not boiling.

2. Pour into a blender and carefully blend on low until frothy.

GLUTEN FREE, NUT FREE, VEGAN *(use maple syrup)*, DAIRY FREE

mango agua fresca

If sipping on cold fruity drinks is your thing, then this is the beverage for you! Aguas frescas are very popular in Mexico, where they are made from all sorts of sweet and sour fruits, flowers, and seeds. They are incredibly refreshing and delicious. They're also easy to make at home. I love the combination of lime and mango, but I urge you to try your hand at different flavor combos. When it's melon season, I am definitely all about blending up pitchers of watermelon aguas frescas and inviting myself over to my neighbors whose houses have pools! **SERVES 2**

2 fresh mangoes, diced
1½ cups water
1 teaspoon fresh lime juice
Pure maple syrup or honey

FOR SERVING
2 cups ice
2 slices fresh lime, for garnish
2 fresh mint sprigs, for garnish

1. In a blender, combine the mango, water, and lime juice and puree until smooth. Taste and add maple syrup or honey, if needed.

2. Fill each of two glasses with 1 cup ice. Pour the agua fresca over the ice and garnish with the lime and mint. Serve immediately.

GLUTEN FREE, NUT FREE, VEGAN *(use maple syrup)*, DAIRY FREE

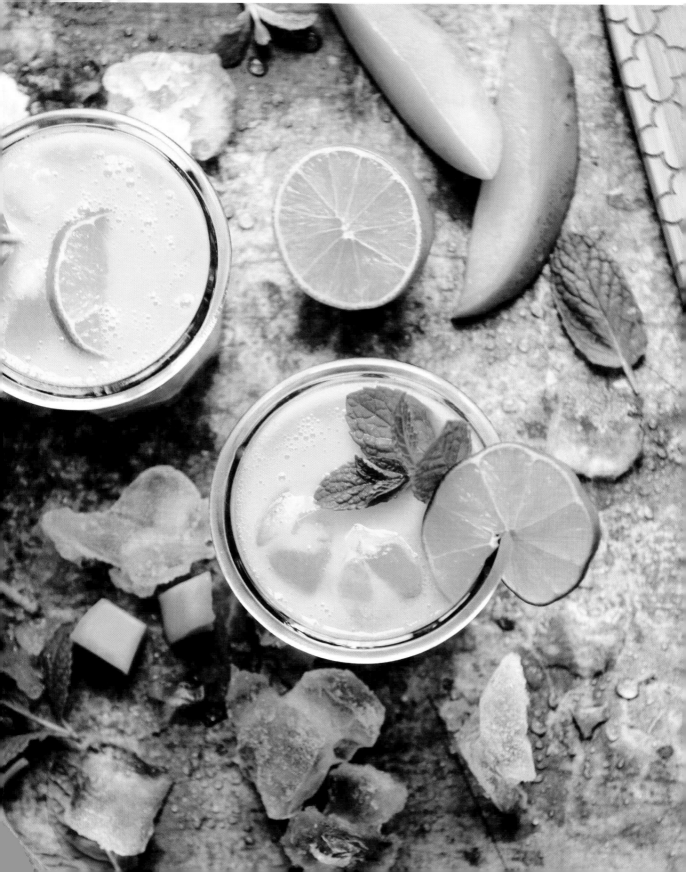

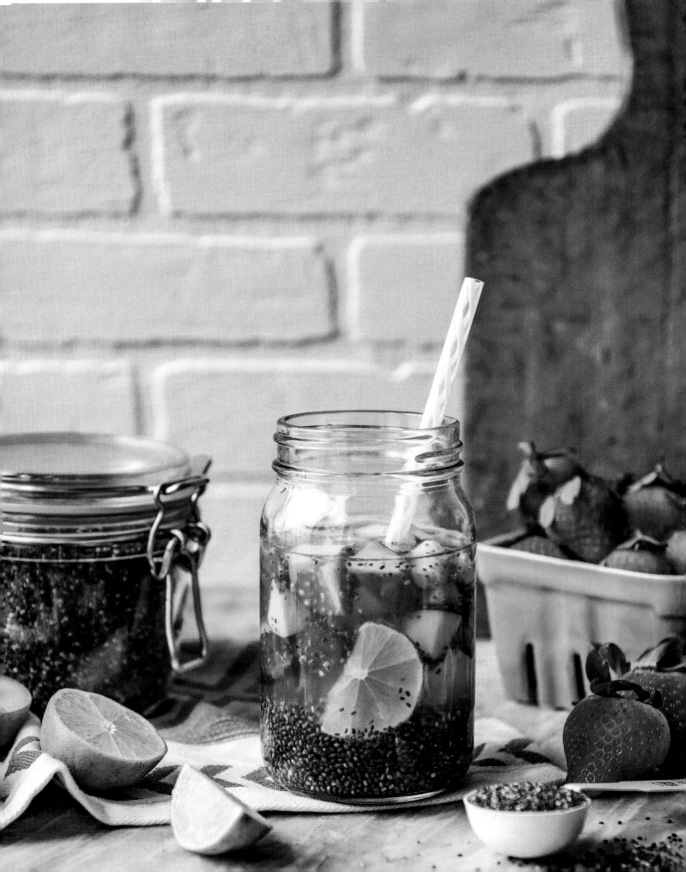

coconut chia fresca

This is truly a natural energy drink if there ever was one! I brought this with me to keep me energized on my 50-K and 100-K ultramarathons in central Florida, and it didn't let me down. Coconut water is full of electrolytes. The chia seeds add protein and healthy fats for a burst of energy, and they also aid digestion. Give this beverage a quick stir before drinking to distribute the seeds, or sip it through a straw and enjoy the little "pop" from the chia seeds—then spoon up all those yummy chunks of fruit at the bottom! **SERVES 1**

1 cup unsweetened coconut water
1 tablespoon chia seeds
1 tablespoon fresh lime juice

½ teaspoon pure maple syrup
¼ cup diced peaches
¼ cup strawberries

1. In a glass or jar, combine the coconut water, chia seeds, lime juice, maple syrup, peaches, and strawberries. Let stand for 5 to 10 minutes, or until the chia seeds absorb some of the liquid and the fruits infuse the water.

2. Refrigerate until ready to drink. Best served chilled. Make sure to enjoy the fruit once you're done sipping the drink!

GLUTEN FREE, NUT FREE, VEGAN, DAIRY FREE

simple hot chocolate

Healthy hot chocolate—is that even possible? It is now! Ditch that packaged stuff and give this version a try. It's incredibly easy to make in the blender (and I've even been known to toss in some spinach leaves, too!). Plus did I mention that it's super chocolatey? Well it is, and my chocolate-loving sweetheart gives it a big thumbs-up. **SERVES 2**

2 tablespoons cacao powder
2 tablespoons pure maple syrup
1 teaspoon pure vanilla extract

Pinch of sea salt
2 cups unsweetened plain almond milk

1. In a small saucepan, whisk together the cacao powder, maple syrup, vanilla, and salt. If you wish to incorporate other flavorings, add them now.

2. Slowly pour the almond milk into the pan, whisking continuously. Keep whisking until the cacao is completely combined.

3. Heat gently over medium heat, whisking occasionally, until hot. Transfer to heatproof mugs and serve immediately.

GLUTEN FREE, NUT FREE *(replace almond milk with coconut milk)*, VEGAN, DAIRY FREE

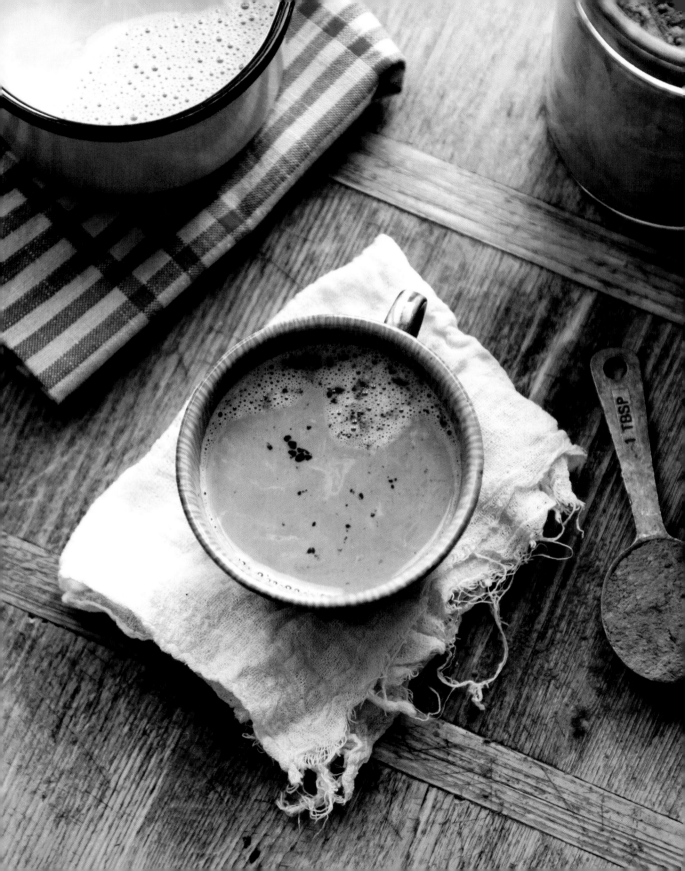

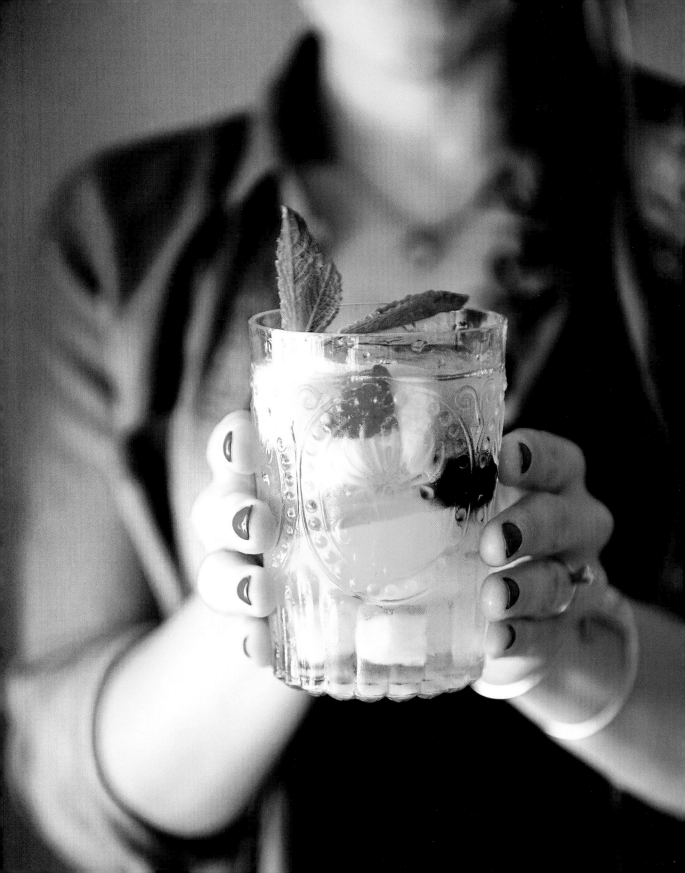

summer sangria

When I was a little girl, my sister and I would throw tea parties for our stuffed animals and serve Kool-Aid in a teapot. Not much has changed, except now I throw game nights with my girlfriends and we serve virgin sangria in adorable wooden pitchers from Target. **SERVES 8**

1 orange, very thinly sliced
1 green apple, cored and thinly sliced
1 ripe-firm white peach, thinly sliced
1 lemon, thinly sliced
1 lime, thinly sliced
1 pint raspberries

1 pint blackberries
1 quart white grape juice
1 bottle (750 ml) sparkling water, chilled

FOR SERVING
Crushed ice
Fresh mint sprigs

1. In a 1-gallon pitcher or beverage container, combine the orange, apple, peach, lemon, lime, raspberries, and blackberries. Pour the grape juice over the fruit. Refrigerate for a few hours, until the fruit flavors infuse the juice.

2. Just before serving, add the sparkling water to the pitcher and stir. Fill 8 glasses with ice and pour sangria over the top. Transfer some of the fruit into the glasses, if desired, and garnish with mint sprigs.

GLUTEN FREE, NUT FREE, VEGAN, DAIRY FREE

rawkstar tip

Use organic fruit to reduce the amount of pesticides and waxes in the sangria or peel fruit to help as well.

autumn spiced cider

Nothing says fall quite like apple cider—and this version takes it to the next level with flavor. Using a slow cooker makes preparing this hot beverage easier than ever, and as the cider mulls, your house will smell fantastic! **MAKES 16 SERVINGS**

1 gallon apple cider
4 whole cinnamon sticks
½ teaspoon ground nutmeg

1 tablespoon whole cloves
1-inch piece fresh ginger, sliced
Peel of 1 organic orange

1. In a slow cooker, combine the cider, cinnamon sticks, nutmeg, cloves, ginger, and orange peel. Heat on low for 8 hours or high for 4 hours, or until the spices infuse the cider. The longer the cider cooks, the stronger the spice flavor will be.

2. Discard the cinnamon sticks, cloves, ginger, and orange peel before serving. Extra cider can be stored in an airtight container for up to 2 weeks in the fridge.

GLUTEN FREE, NUT FREE, VEGAN, DAIRY FREE

rawkstar tip

To make it easier to remove the spices and peel, place them in a few layers of cheesecloth and tie with string to make a nice little bundle. For a sweeter sip, add honey or maple syrup.

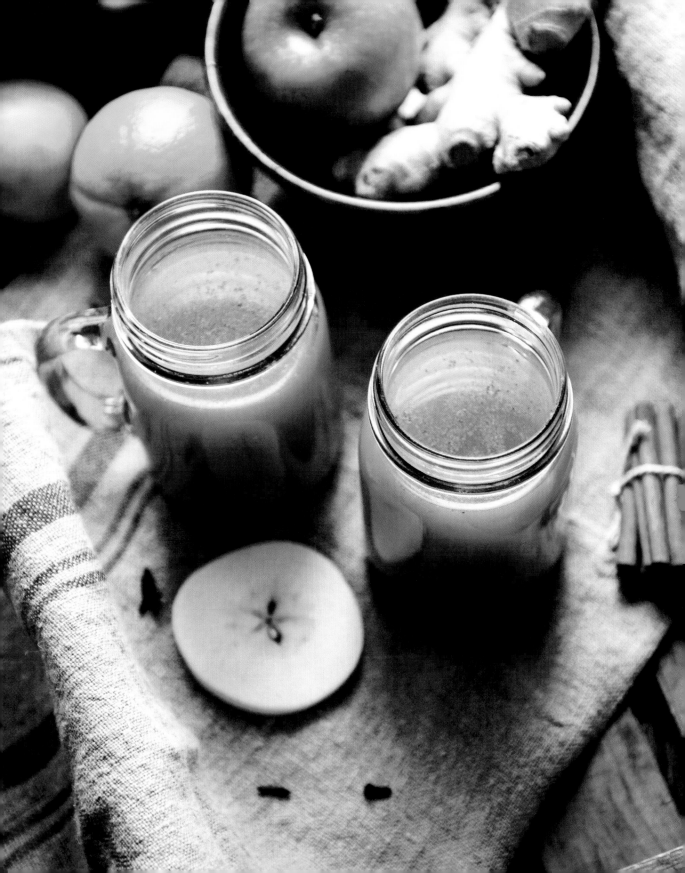

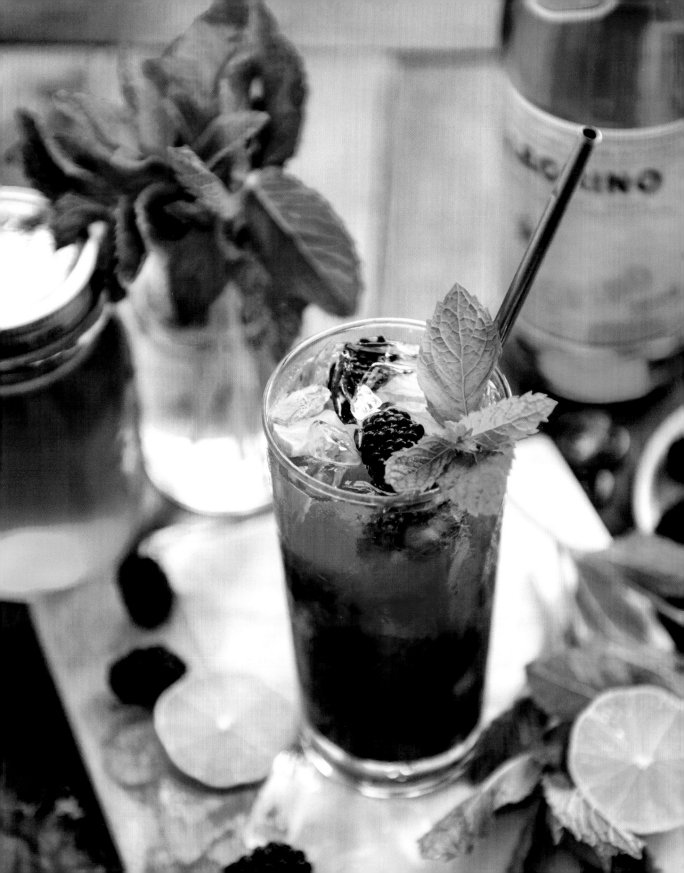

blackberry mojito

I know you're going to love this virgin take on a classic summer party drink. It's light, refreshing, and makes me think I'm on "island time." The blackberries ramp up the fresh flavor and give this beverage a pretty purple hue. Of course, you could leave them out for the classic drink, but think of all the healthful antioxidants you'd be missing out on! **SERVES 2**

¼ cup water
¼ cup organic cane sugar
10 fresh mint leaves
1 cup blackberries

1 lime, quartered
2 cups crushed ice
16 ounces sparkling water

1. In a small saucepan, combine the water and sugar. Bring to a simmer over medium-high heat, stirring occasionally, to dissolve the sugar. Stop stirring and let the mixture boil for 1 minute. Remove from the heat and let cool completely.

2. Place 4 mint leaves, ½ cup of the blackberries, and 2 lime quarters in each of 2 large glasses. Using a muddler or the end of a wooden spoon, squash the mint, berries, and limes 10 times to release the juice and flavor.

3. Add half of the sugar water to each glass. Stir a little bit, then add 1 cup ice to each glass. Pour 8 ounces of the sparkling water over the top. Garnish with the extra mint leaves and lime quarters. Serve immediately.

GLUTEN FREE, NUT FREE, VEGAN, DAIRY FREE

energizing tea latte

It's hard for me to comprehend, but not everyone loves coffee like I do. No joke, I am the coffee junkie who once looked deep into a barista's eyes and begged her to create an IV drip of caffeine just for me. I've come a long way since then. I actually started expanding my warm beverage offerings when we have tea-loving friends over—and this simple tea latte is always on the menu. **SERVES 1**

1 cup unsweetened cashew milk
2 teaspoons raw honey
½ teaspoon pure vanilla extract

1½ teaspoons matcha powder
¼ cup boiling water

1. In a small saucepan, heat the cashew milk over medium heat for 3 to 5 minutes or until very hot but not boiling. Stir in the honey and vanilla.

2. Place the matcha powder into a mug and whisk in the boiling water to make a paste. For a frothy texture, place the milk in a blender and blend for 10 seconds on high, or use a whisk to froth the milk by hand. Pour the milk into the mug with the matcha tea, adding any foam to the top. Drink immediately.

VARIATION

For an iced latte: Whisk the matcha powder with the boiling water to make a paste. Let cool slightly. Stir in the vanilla and 2 tablespoons of cashew milk. The mixture should be pourable. Fill a tall glass with crushed ice and add the matcha mixture. Fill the glass to the top with the remaining milk. Drink immediately.

GLUTEN FREE, NUT FREE *(swap cashew milk with coconut milk)*, VEGAN *(use maple syrup instead of honey)*, DAIRY FREE

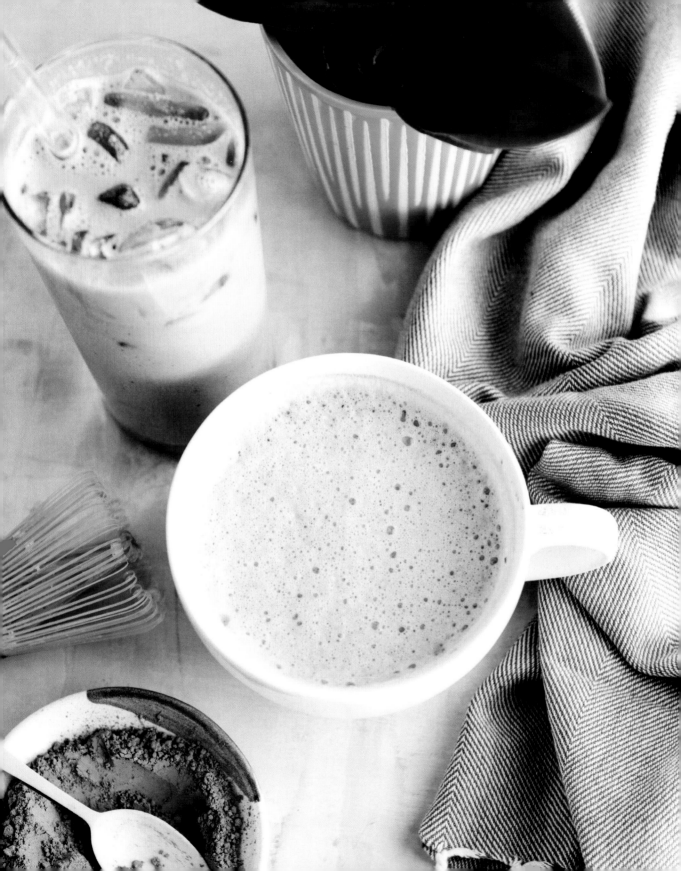

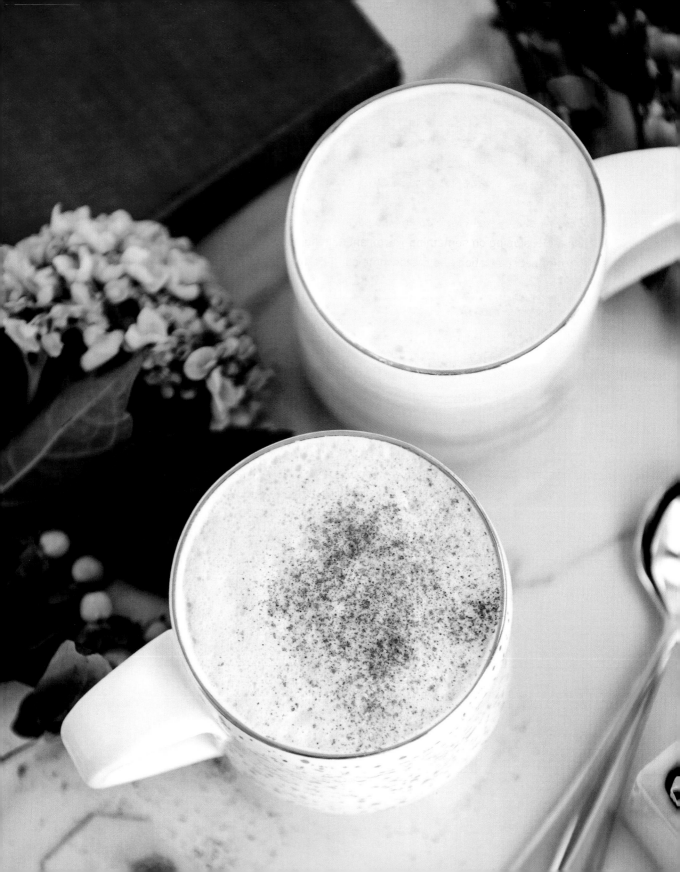

vanilla steamer

Ryan and I have always sat at the breakfast table to enjoy our coffee in the morning, and—before this recipe—the kids would inevitably ask for a sip. We let them, time and time again, have a swig of java, and of course they couldn't stand it. They would spit it out and complain, "How can you drink that?!" Yet they made the request again and again. Eventually, I realized what they really wanted: to be a part of the experience of sitting around the kitchen table, sipping on something warm, and talking about the day ahead. This recipe arose from that realization and has become our kids' favorite morning beverage while we drink our coffee. **SERVES 1**

1 cup unsweetened plain almond milk
2 teaspoons pure maple syrup

½ teaspoon pure vanilla extract
Pinch of ground cinnamon

1. In a small saucepan over medium heat, warm the almond milk for 5 minutes, or until very hot but not boiling.

2. Transfer the hot milk to a blender, then add the maple syrup and vanilla. Carefully blend on low speed for 10 seconds, then increase the speed to high and blend until frothy and well combined.

3. Pour into a heatproof mug, sprinkle with cinnamon, and enjoy immediately.

GLUTEN FREE, NUT FREE *(replace almond milk with coconut milk)*, VEGAN, DAIRY FREE

simple sodas

When you embrace a plant-powered life and try to avoid processed foods, sodas are one of the first things to go. This recipe is a fabulous way to bring back "soda" in a nutritious way. My kids still don't like carbonated beverages, but as they get older and their tastes change, I know what we will be making first! **SERVES 1**

STRAWBERRY-VANILLA

1 cup organic cane sugar
1 cup water
1½ cups strawberries
1 vanilla bean, split lengthwise

PEACH-ROSEMARY

1 cup organic cane sugar
1 cup water
1½ cups chopped peaches
Sprig of rosemary

LAVENDER-BLUEBERRY-LEMON

1 cup organic cane sugar
1 cup water
1½ cups blueberries, fresh or frozen
3 tablespoons fresh lemon juice
1 teaspoon dried culinary lavender buds

MANGO-JALAPEÑO

1 cup organic cane sugar
1 cup water
1½ cups chopped mango
2 tablespoons fresh lime juice
½ jalapeño chile pepper, sliced

1. Choose a flavor. Place the sugar, water, fruit, and any other ingredients in a saucepan. Bring to a boil, then reduce the heat to low and simmer for about 20 minutes, or until the fruit has released its juices and is very, very soft.

2. Strain the syrup though a fine-mesh sieve to remove seeds, peels, and other solids. There should be about 2 cups of syrup. Allow to cool, then transfer to a jar with a tight-fitting lid and store in the refrigerator for up to 2 weeks, or freeze for several months until ready to use.

3. *To make soda:* Add 3 tablespoons of the strained syrup to 1 cup sparkling water. Serve chilled or over ice.

GLUTEN FREE, NUT FREE, VEGAN, DAIRY FREE

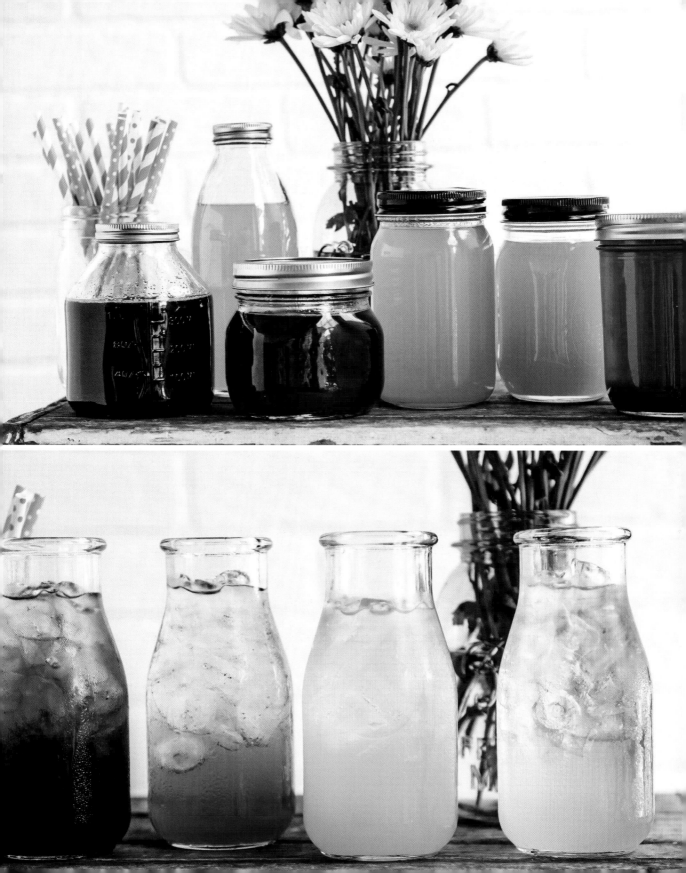

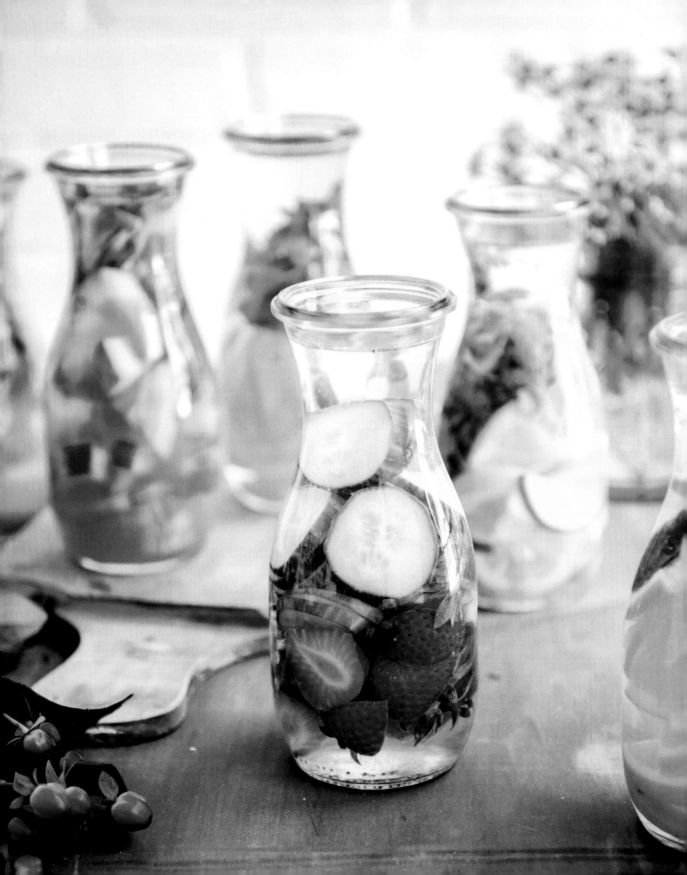

fruit-infused coolers

One of the easiest ways to become a healthier person is to simply drink more water. I know how boring that can be, so it doesn't always happen. To help me get excited to chug the H_2O, I often doctor it up with a bit of fresh fruit and herbs. **SERVES 1**

PINEAPPLE MINT

½ cup chopped pineapple
5 mint leaves
2 cups filtered water

MANGO BASIL

½ cup chopped and seeded mango
5 basil leaves
2 cups filtered water

STRAWBERRY CUCUMBER

½ organic cucumber, sliced
3 organic strawberries
2 cups filtered water

WATERMELON BASIL

½ cup chopped watermelon
5 basil leaves
2 cups filtered water

TRIPLE CITRUS CILANTRO

1 organic orange, sliced
½ organic lemon, sliced
½ organic lime, sliced
2 tablespoons chopped cilantro
2 cups filtered water

ORANGE CINNAMON

1 organic orange, sliced
1 cinnamon stick
2 cups filtered water

1. Choose a flavor. In a quart mason jar or carafe, combine the fruit, herbs, and spices.

2. Fill the jar with the filtered water. Place in the fridge for 30 minutes or longer, until the flavors infuse. The fruit-infused coolers will keep for several days in the fridge. The water can be replenished 1 or 2 times, but the flavor may not be as strong.

GLUTEN FREE, NUT FREE, VEGAN, DAIRY FREE

soothing tea tonic

Since 2011, our family has been able to say "no thank you" to cold and flu medications—no Tylenol, Zicam, DayQuil, antibiotics, you name it. We use whole foods, homeopathy, rest, and hot showers to heal our bodies from the inside out. Medicine has a place—yet I think we often use it before we've given nutrition and nature a chance. I've come to rely on this simple DIY remedy when cold and flu season hits our family. It quickly soothes itchy throats, reduces congestion, settles upset tummies, and relaxes achy bodies. **SERVES 8**

2 organic lemons, sliced
2-inch piece fresh ginger, peeled and sliced

1 cup raw honey, plus more as needed

1. In a mason jar with a lid, stack the lemon and ginger slices in alternating layers. Slowly pour in some of the honey. Allow the honey to sink down and around the lemon and ginger, then add more honey. Once you have filled the jar to the top, attach the lid and seal tightly. Store in the refrigerator. Over time, the mixture will start to turn into a loose jelly.

2. When you are in need of some soothing tea, spoon 2 tablespoons into a mug full of hot water—be sure to scoop up whole pieces of ginger and lemon. Steep for 3 minutes and sip away.

GLUTEN FREE, NUT FREE, DAIRY FREE

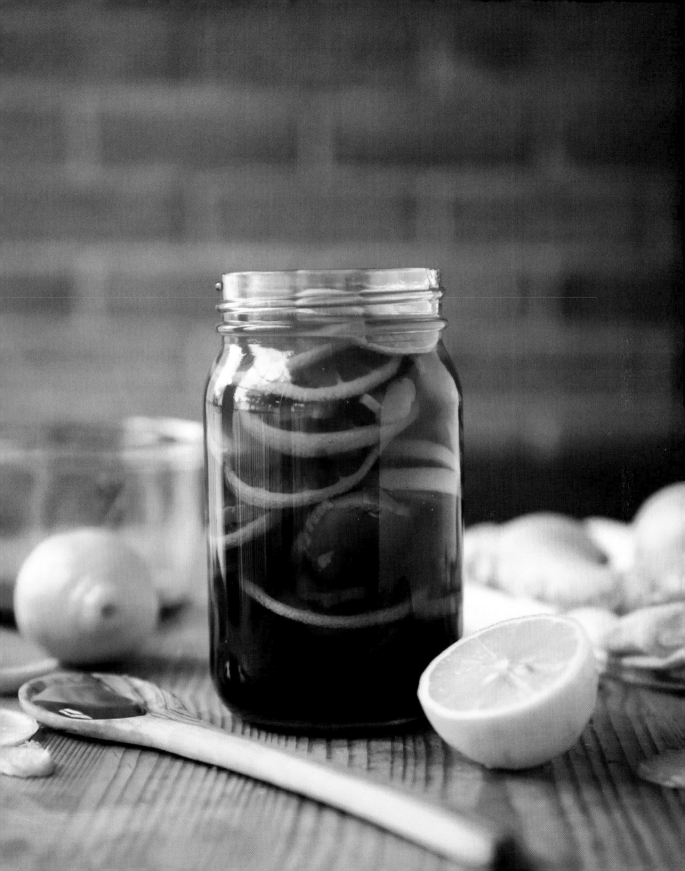

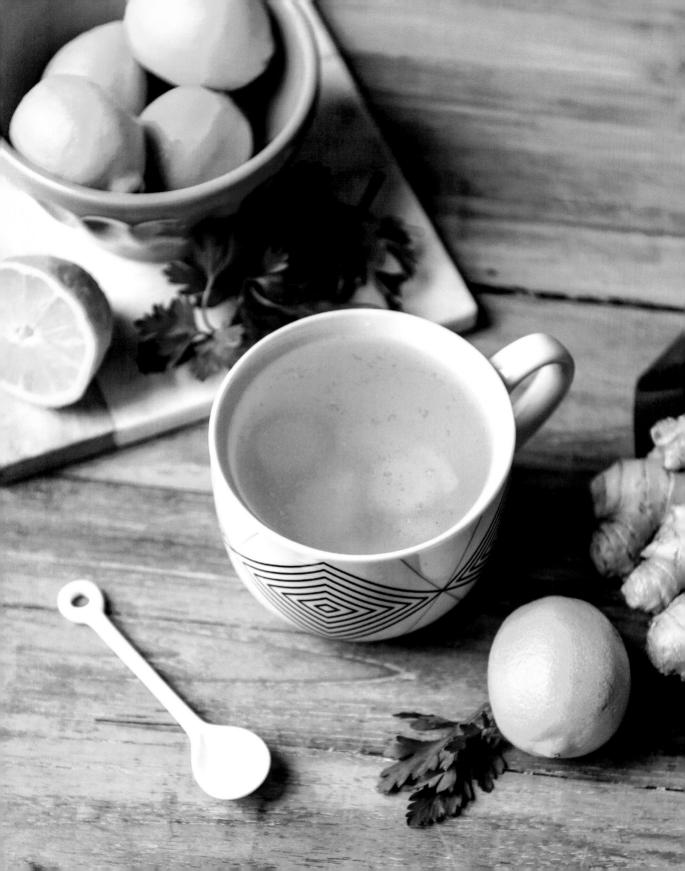

fresh start morning tonic

One of the best things you can do for your digestive system is to start each morning with hot water and lemon. This is a vital part of our 21-day cleanse program, Fresh Start (http://sgs.to/cleanse). The lemon promotes alkalinity in the body and also kick-starts the liver for the day—encouraging the release of digestive fluids. Add in ground red pepper and fresh ginger to bring warmth to the tummy and boost your metabolism and circulation. Parsley is an optional add-in that will tack on extra alkalinity and nutrients to your morning routine. **SERVES 1**

1 cup water
1-inch piece fresh ginger, thinly sliced
1 tablespoon fresh lemon juice

Pinch of ground red pepper (optional)
1 teaspoon fresh parsley (optional)

1. Bring the water to a boil in a saucepan or kettle. Place the ginger and lemon juice in a mug, pour in the hot water, and allow it to steep for 5 minutes.

2. Add the red pepper and parsley, if using, and enjoy immediately.

GLUTEN FREE, NUT FREE, DAIRY FREE

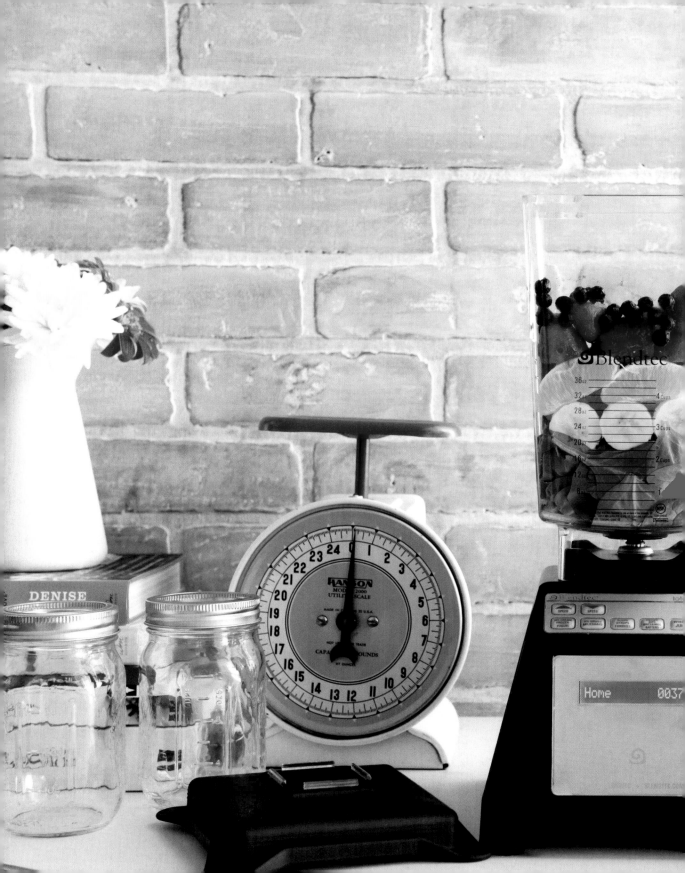

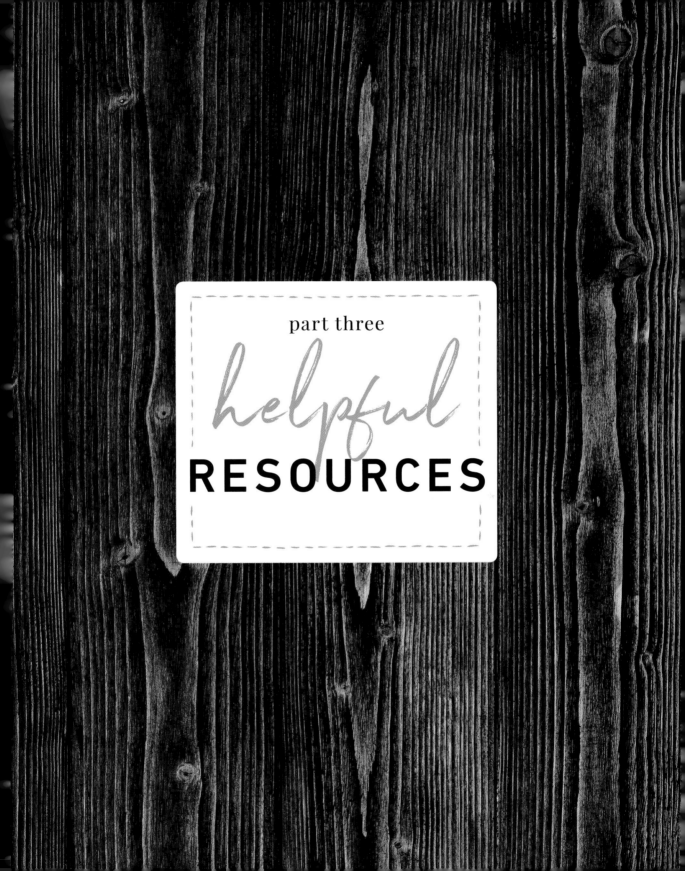

part three

helpful

RESOURCES

PROTEIN SOURCES
plant-based power

Did you know that pound for pound, kale actually contains more protein than red meat? It's true! Now while it may also be true that you can eat a steak and get your protein faster than eating a pound of greens, there's also all that red meat's saturated fat and zero dietary fiber to consider. Not to mention it is incredibly hard on the body to digest animal protein. The nutrients in plant-based foods are absorbed much more readily in the body than nutrients from meat.

Okay, does this mean you have to stop eating meat? No, but you probably could benefit from adding more leafy greens, beans and legumes, root veggies, fruit, and healthy whole grains to your lifestyle. Here's a list of plants that are highest in protein.

SEEDS AND GRAINS

NAME	SERVING SIZE	PROTEIN CONTENT
Quinoa	1 cup	24 grams
Pumpkin seeds	½ cup	19.5 grams
Cacao powder	1 cup	17 grams
Nutritional yeast	¼ cup	16 grams

NUTS

NAME	SERVING SIZE	PROTEIN CONTENT
Almond butter	¼ cup	16 grams
Macadamia nuts	1 cup	10.6 grams
Hemp seeds	3 T	9 grams
Almonds and walnuts, whole	¼ cup	8 grams
Pecans, whole	¼ cup	5 grams

LEGUMES

NAME	SERVING SIZE	PROTEIN CONTENT
Lentils, cooked	1 cup	18 grams
Black beans	1 cup	15.24 grams
Cannellini beans	1 cup	15.3 grams
Chickpeas	1 cup	14.53 grams
Kidney beans	1 cup	7.73 grams

VEGETABLES

NAME	SERVING SIZE	PROTEIN CONTENT
Dulse	1 cup	10 grams
Arugula	1 cup	5.16 grams
Portobello mushrooms	1 cup	5 grams
Asparagus	1 cup	4.32 grams

FRUITS

NAME	SERVING SIZE	PROTEIN CONTENT
Avocado	1	4.02 grams
Thai coconut	1 cup	2.7 grams
Plantain	1	2.33 grams
Apricots	1 cup	2.31 grams
Kiwifruit	1 cup	2.05 grams

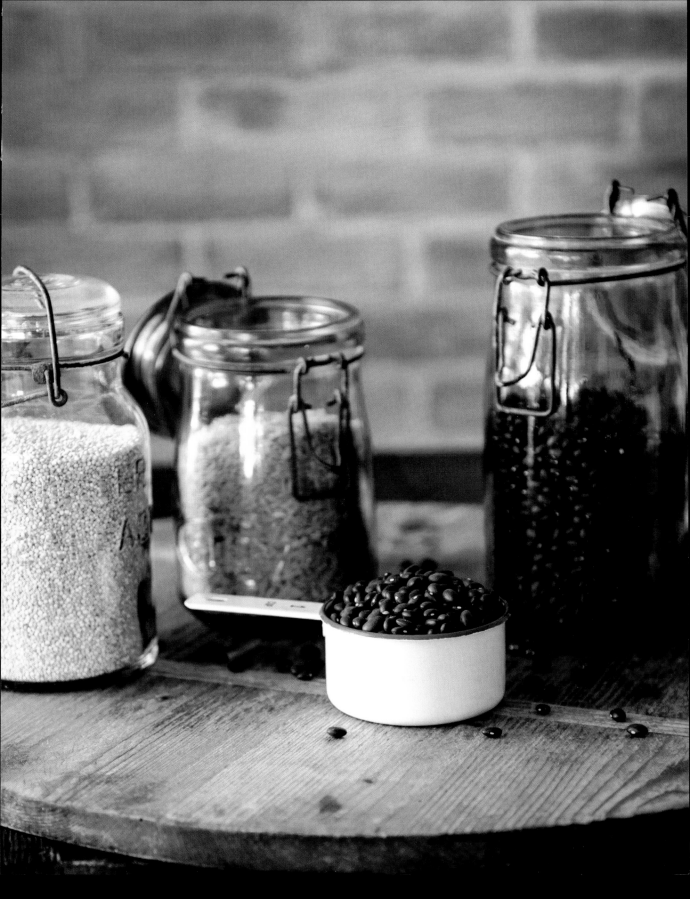

EGG REPLACERS
fun with edible chemistry

Eggs are a great source of protein and have become a staple in our house since we started raising eight hens and Huck the Duck a few years ago. Most of the recipes in this book are vegan and gluten-free, yet occasionally we bring an egg to the party. If you'd rather not consume eggs, you can still make our recipes by following these replacement tips grouped by the role eggs will be fulfilling in your recipe: leavening, binding, or adding moisture.

LEAVENING

In baked goods—such as cakes, cookies, pies, and bread—eggs encourage ingredients to ferment and rise. These alternatives will bring about the same or similar fluffy result.

1. **APPLE CIDER VINEGAR**. It seems the list of uses for apple cider vinegar never ends. In this case, combine 1 tablespoon apple cider vinegar with 1 teaspoon baking soda to create a leavening agent.

2. **CARBONATED WATER**. Possibly the easiest leavening substitute is carbonated water, if you have it on hand (which I never seem to). Simply replace ¼ cup of the liquid ingredients with carbonated water. For example, if making a pancake recipe that calls for 1 cup almond milk and 1 egg, just omit the egg and use ¾ cup almond milk and ¼ cup carbonated water.

3. **BAKING POWDER**. Mix 2 tablespoons water with 1 tablespoon of your choice of oil and 2 tablespoons baking powder to replace 1 egg.

BINDING

Since eggs harden as they are heated, they hold the ingredients together in a recipe. When you have a recipe that already contains a leavening agent such as baking powder, baking soda, or vinegar, you can use the following to substitute as a binding agent:

1. **MASHED BANANA OR AVOCADO**. Half a medium-size mashed banana or ¼ cup mashed avocado can replace an egg. These options are best used in cookies, brownies, and pancakes. However, don't use an overripe banana—the flavor can overpower the recipe.

2. **CHIA SEEDS**. Wisk together 1 tablespoon ground chia seeds with 3 tablespoons water and let soak for 10 minutes to create a sticky, gelatinous texture to replace 1 egg.

3. **FLAXSEEDS**. Similarly, wisk together 1 tablespoon ground flaxseeds with 3 tablespoons water and let soak for 10 minutes to create a sticky, gelatinous texture to replace 1 egg.

4. **NUT BUTTER**. Three tablespoons nut butter can replace 1 egg. This option is best used in cookies, brownies, or pancakes. Be sure to use the creamy, not chunky, nut butter for a smooth texture.

MOISTENING

Eggs are a liquid and full of fat, so these replacers can do the job of making your recipes rich and moist.

1. **APPLESAUCE**. One egg can be replaced by ¼ cup of applesauce.

2. **PUMPKIN PUREE**. In addition to replacing an egg, pumpkin puree also adds flavor. Try it in pumpkin bread, muffins, or pancakes by simply adding ¼ cup to replace 1 egg.

SOAKING NUTS AND SEEDS

Soaking nuts and seeds helps remove and break down any "antinutrients" like enzyme inhibitors, lectins, phytates, and tannins, plus soaking creates a creamier result for recipes where the nuts are blended or food processed. The soaking process is particularly helpful for those who need to be extra gentle on their tummies when it comes to digestion. At the same time, you're helping your body absorb the vitamins and minerals more easily. You may notice that your stomach is just fine digesting raw nuts and seeds, and if that's the case, and the recipe doesn't require soaking, feel free to skip!

HOW TO SOAK

1. Add nuts or seeds to a glass bowl, pour room-temperature filtered water over them, and cover the bowl with a towel (to allow it to breathe) while they soak. Follow a 2:1 ratio of 2 parts water to 1 part nuts or seeds. For example: 2 cups water and 1 cup almonds. You can add a squeeze of lemon juice to help break down the nuts' enzyme inhibitors.

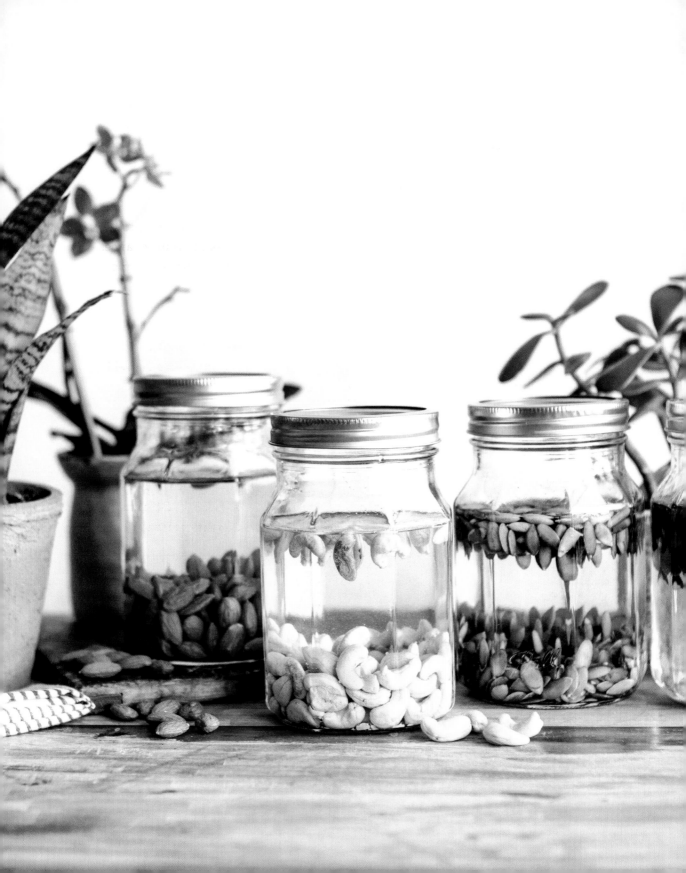

2. After the nuts or seeds have soaked for their recommended time (see the chart), drain the water, rinse, and add them to your recipe. Make sure to give some extra rinse love: Rinse until the water appears clear.

SOAKING TIMES FOR NUTS AND SEEDS

8+ HOURS
Almonds
Flaxseeds
Hazelnuts
Macadamia nuts
Pumpkin seeds
Sesame seeds

4–8 HOURS
Brazil nuts
Pecans
Pistachio nuts
Walnuts

2–4 HOURS
Cashews
Sunflower seeds

DON'T SOAK
Hemp seeds
Pine nuts

Pssst . . . You can soak nuts up to 2 days at room temperature (a good thing in case you forget about that bowl of nuts on your counter—I've totally done this).

HOW TO SPEED SOAK NUTS

If you're short on time or simply forgot to soak your nuts or seeds in advance. I've got a shortcut that has saved me many times. Yet it's important to note that this shortcut does destroy the raw nuts' live enzymes and zaps their nutritional value. So I don't recommend making this your default method of soaking, but it can help in a pinch.

1. Place the nuts in a bowl. Boil enough water to cover the nuts by an inch.

2. Pour the boiling water over the nuts and let soak for 30 minutes or longer (depending on the nut).

3. Drain and rinse. Then you're ready to go!

PACK YOUR PANTRY, FILL YOUR FRIDGE

This handy-dandy produce storing guide will help you stop wondering where to put the garlic or the ginger.

FRESH FRUITS

APPLE: Store away from vegetables, as apples produce ethylene, a ripening agent.

AVOCADO: Ripen avocados in a paper bag on the countertop. When fully ripe, eat quickly.

BANANA: Store on the countertop and don't refrigerate, as this stops the ripening process and turns the skin brown.

BLUEBERRIES: Store in the coldest part of the refrigerator, loosely covered with plastic wrap. Do not wash until ready to use, because fresh berries are highly perishable.

CUCUMBER: Keep refrigerated.

GRAPES: Keep grapes attached to the stem and they should last in the fridge for 3 to 5 days. Do not wash until ready to use.

LEMON: Store away from other fruits to avoid absorption of offensive flavors, and wash before using.

LIME: Store away from other fruits to avoid absorption of offensive flavors, and wash before using.

MANGO: Keep refrigerated.

NECTARINES: Keep refrigerated.

ORANGES: Store on the countertop, and always refrigerate cut citrus.

PEACHES: Keep refrigerated.

PEARS: Keep refrigerated.

PINEAPPLE: Store on the countertop, and always refrigerate cut pineapple.

RASPBERRIES: Store in the coldest part of the refrigerator, loosely covered with plastic wrap. Do not wash until you are ready to use, because fresh berries are highly perishable.

STRAWBERRIES: Store in the coldest part of the refrigerator, loosely covered with plastic wrap. Do not wash until you are ready to use, because fresh strawberries are highly perishable.

DRIED FRUITS

APRICOTS: Store in the pantry or refrigerator.

CRANBERRIES: Store in the pantry or refrigerator.

FIGS: Store in the pantry or refrigerator.

GOJI BERRIES: Store in the pantry or refrigerator.

VEGETABLES

BEETS: Cut the leaves 2 inches from the root, bag the leaves and root separately, and refrigerate.

BELL PEPPERS: Store in a container or bag in the refrigerator.

BROCCOLI: Store in a container or bag in the refrigerator.

BUTTERNUT SQUASH: Store in a cool, dry place, and do not refrigerate.

CABBAGE: Store in a perforated plastic bag, away from fruits, to avoid deterioration.

CARROTS: Remove the tops and store in a perforated plastic bag.

CAULIFLOWER: Store in a container or bag in the refrigerator.

CELERY: Keep refrigerated in a perforated plastic bag.

CHERRY TOMATOES: Do not refrigerate, as it will make the tomatoes mealy and flavorless.

CHIVES: Place in a container or bag in the refrigerator.

FENNEL: Place in a container or bag in the refrigerator.

GARLIC: Keep at room temperature.

GINGER: Wrap in a paper towel and store in a paper bag in the refrigerator.

KALE: Store in a perforated plastic bag, away from fruits, to avoid deterioration.

LEEKS: Cut off and discard the dark green tops; place in a container or bag in the refrigerator.

OLIVES: Store in the refrigerator in an airtight container.

ONION: Store in a cool, dry area.

PEAS: Store in a bag in the refrigerator for a couple days, as they do not have a long shelf life.

POTATO: Store in a cool, dark place, like the bottom of the pantry.

PUMPKIN: Once opened, refrigerate canned pumpkin in an airtight container.

SCALLIONS: Cut off the roots, place in a container or bag, and put in the refrigerator.

SPINACH: Store in a perforated plastic bag, away from fruits, to avoid deterioration.

SWEET POTATOES: Store in a cool, dry place with good ventilation, but do not refrigerate.

TOMATOES: Do not refrigerate, as it will make the tomatoes mealy and flavorless.

ZUCCHINI: Refrigerate in a plastic bag.

HERBS

HERBS: Wash and dry them, snip off the stem ends and submerge the stems in a glass of water or set in water like flowers, cover with a plastic bag, and leave in the refrigerator.

ACKNOWLEDGMENTS

MY LOVES

Ryan, thanks for believing in me and supporting me every step of the way. Saying yes to that first date 19 years ago was the best decision of my life. I will always choose you, again and again. We have many adventures ahead of us, and I promise to love you through them all.

Jackson, I don't know how you are so mature for being only 10, but you are. Thank you for understanding when I have to go away to write and then celebrating with me when I come home. All your advice during the recipe testing has made these recipes a thousand times better. Kids around the world can thank you for that. You are a top chef in the making.

Clare, you truly light a room up when you walk in. Thank you for making me smile daily and giving the best hugs after long days of writing. Your own passion for eating healthy and moving your body is going to change the world—keep showing up just as you are.

MY FAMILY

Dad, Mom, Steph, Mike, Amanda, and Joe, I couldn't ask for a better family. I am beyond blessed by every single one of you. You speak truth, love big, and will catch me when I fall—you make me a better person every day.

John, Debi, Candice, and Dave, taking on the Hansard name is an honor, and I'm thankful to have married into your family. Thank you for accepting me as I am.

Mi familia de iglesia, muchas gracias para su amor y apoya. ¡Les amo mucho! Un dia voy a tener un libro de espanol especialmente para nosotros. Dios de bendiga—the Rojas, Padillas, Amazons, and Laras.

Thanks Brooksville Wesleyan Church for your support to allow me to pursue my passions inside and outside the church walls.

To the Gromans, Sweeneys, Desnoyers, Hansards, and Laws: I love you all! I truly have the best family. Thank you for always being here for our family and for me—your love is felt daily, and your prayers have protected us and blessed my family. I hope this book is a blessing to you, too.

To my friends who call, text, come beside me, and pray at the perfect times to support me in many small but powerful ways: Carissa Vanderford, Kaley Moore, Jen Johnston, Rachelle Gilmore, Lori Benefiel, Erin Mottayaw, Dilma Samayoa, Kathleen Borozny, Katie Vandermead, the Styers family, Jenni Reichart, Andrea Baker, the Harmons, Trish Tice, and the Pence family.

MY RAWKSTAR FAMILY

Dan Mottayaw, you're a great leader, and I couldn't and wouldn't have wanted to go through these past few years without you. Thank you for sharing so many great ideas and taking action on them to make Simple Green Smoothies what it is today.

Lindsey Johnson, your passion for cooking and talent for food photography are remarkable. You brought this beautiful book to life, and I'm so thankful for all that you've brought to Simple Green Smoothies.

Amanda Frisbie, your excitement for our community breathes life into Simple Green Smoothies every single day. Thank you for saying yes again and again as we have grown into a magnificent company.

Liz and Ryan Bower, you came into my life at just the right time. Your tech skills and creative talents blow my mind and have been so valuable to the company and my sanity.

Kim Wester, you have kept me going. Your support and positivity through it all has meant so much to me.

Nikki Klukowski, you came on board as our rawkstar intern, and I threw you into this book with me. Thank you for going 90 mph with me. You are an incredible writer, and the world needs your voice in it.

Jessie Provience, thank you for being the most generous, passionate person I have ever met. Your desire to make the world a better place inspires me daily.

Tessa Brennan, the courageous talent inside of you is unreal! I am so thankful you shared it with Simple Green Smoothies. You will always be our rawkstar.

Jadah Sellner, Simple Green Smoothies will always have a piece of you in it. Thanks for dreaming with me back in 2012.

Meg Thompson, your passion for whole foods has become my passion. Thank you for opening my world to quinoa, buckwheat, hemp hearts, and so many more incredible plant-powered foods.

The Rawkstar community, thank you for testing these recipes to turn them from good to great. This book wouldn't be half as good without you: Courtney Anderson, Sarah Andrews, Karen Arban, Keah Archie-King, Katie Baker, Samantha Bengel, Nancy Blue, Shelli Boer, Susan Boissonneault, Meridith Braun, Alie Bultman, Jessica Burns, Carlina Capelo-Pichardo, Kristina Carigiet, Kelsey Carter, Susan Chapman, Angelica Chimal, Ozlem Cigeroglu, Stephanie Conant, Jamee Cordell, Olivia Cox, Jenny De La Loza, Kayleen Diederich, Jennifer Donald, Carmen Fischer, Shannon Frey, Sheri Fry, Rebecca Gerity, Rhonda Gibler, Samantha Gilbane, Connie Gordon,

Maya Greenfield, Anita Hains, Alita Hanley, Jacky Hansen, Elizabeth Higgins, Kathy Hildin, Merel Homan, Toni Jakes, Ana Lia Johnson, Kate LaGrand Nienhuis, Stephanie Malmstrom, Paula Mariani, Cynda Marrufo, Beth Mastroianni, Susan May, Mimi McBride, Elysa McDonald, Janis McGuffin, Alison McKenzie, Julia Mönks, Genevieve Morehead, Kim Morosco, Joanna Nelson, Andrea Nestvold, Carolyn Oates, Jennifer Olson, Taryn Olson, Heather O'Sullivan, Jen Paleracio, Sara Pereira, Paige Peterson, Anastasia Peuhkurinen, Lanae Phelps, Lucrece Pierre-Carr, Sarah Pietsch, Katrina Piva, Kerenza Reid, Jennifer Riemer, Marcy Riley, Rachelle Roberts, Sara Rogers, Anna Rose, Stacey Rosenberger, Clarissa Santiago, Gayatri Sathe, Lisa Savage, Anne Schwartz, Emily Seay, Angela Smith, Renee Stewart, Heidi Stoltenburg, Saraswathi Subramanian, Kendra Tassara, Mary Tastsides, Kristin Thornton, Kathy Toding, Cara Toth, Christina Tropiano, Caitlin Varhalla, April Victor, Lakeisha Wall, Sonja Wheatley, Janine White, Alexis Williams, Elizabeth and Grace Williams, Amber Wilson, Connie Wilson, and Michelle Wood.

MY COACHES

Christen Bavero, you helped me find my spark. Thank you for asking the hard questions over and over and giving me a safe space to dream out loud and go after it.

Lane Kennedy, this book is in your hands because of your persistence. Thank you for pushing me and guiding me when things got rocky and I couldn't see through the forest.

MY BOOK TEAM

Rodale, thank you for believing in me. One book was a dream come true; now to have a second is a blessing. You are giving me a larger platform to share my message and change the world. Thanks to the editors, designers, and marketing team who brought this to life, especially Diana Baroni, Michele Eniclerico, Mark McCauslin, Nicole LaRoche, Phil Leung, Gail Gonzales, Jennifer Levesque, Marisa Vigilante, Allison Janice, Danielle Curtis, Christina Foxley, and Brianne Sperber.

Scott Hoffman and Steve Troha, at times I think you believed in my book more than I did. Thank you for the encouragement to keep on going and share my message with the world. You truly are the most caring and passionate book agents in the world, and I'm blessed to call you mine.

My talented photographers, Jim Cook and Ilde Cook—thank you for capturing my family in the most beautiful way. Lindsey Johnson—you took my art direction and ran with it to make the most inspirational recipe photographs of all time.

Hannah Armstrong and Allison Tafelski, thank you for making me feel extra pretty and confident for the photo shoot. Your passion and heart for creativity shine through in these lifestyle images.

Erin Mottayaw, thank you for editing and recipe testing during many phases of this book's evolution. Your swap suggestions are amazing!

SIMPLE GREEN MEAL PLANS

One of the best ways I've found to eat well and keep my sanity is meal planning. I've created 4 weeks of dinner plans and a weekly shopping list to get you started. This will have a family of four covered for an entire month of dinners, while still taking 2 days off a week to allow for leftovers and a night eating out. (You can only cook so much!)

What works best for me is to do my grocery shopping on Saturdays and spend an hour prepping on Sundays. This can include chopping vegetables, cooking rice and quinoa, and even making some meals ahead of time. Sunday prep gives me a little advantage when Monday afternoon rolls around and we've gotta get dinner on the table before we head out the door for an activity.

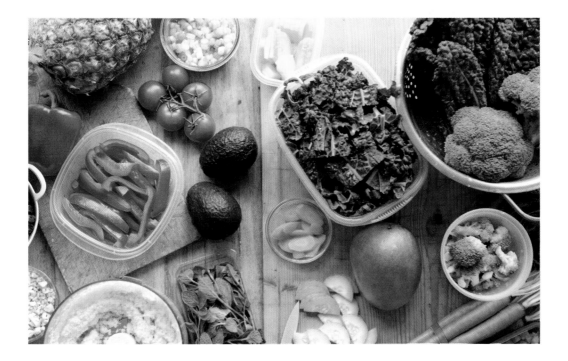

WEEK 1

DAY 1

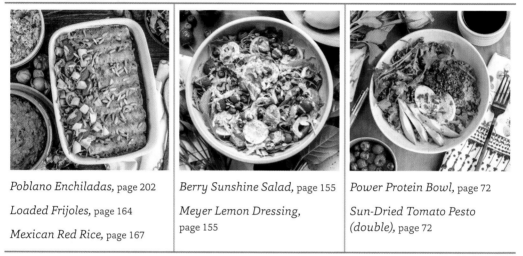

Poblano Enchiladas, page 202

Loaded Frijoles, page 164

Mexican Red Rice, page 167

DAY 2

Berry Sunshine Salad, page 155

Meyer Lemon Dressing, page 155

DAY 3

Power Protein Bowl, page 72

Sun-Dried Tomato Pesto (double), page 72

DAY 4

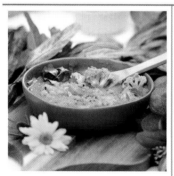

Veggie Lentil Stew, page 190

DAY 5

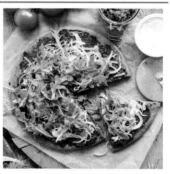

Savory Quinoa Pizza, page 174

shopping list

FRESH FRUIT
1 ripe and 2 green avocados
1 cup blueberries
1 lemon
1 lime
3 Meyer lemons
2 oranges
1 cup raspberries
1 cup strawberries

FRESH VEGETABLES
10 cups baby arugula
1 cup baby kale
1 bunch of basil
2 carrots
3 cups cauliflower
1 cup cherry tomatoes
1 bunch of cilantro
2 fennel bulbs
8 garlic cloves
4 golden potatoes
1 bunch of kale
2 poblano peppers
1 red onion
1 cup romaine lettuce
2 small shallots
1 white onion
1 yellow onion

OILS AND LIQUIDS
avocado oil
virgin coconut oil
4 eggs
extra-virgin olive oil
honey
16 cups vegetable stock

NUTS AND SEEDS
1 cup almonds, raw
1 cup cashews, raw
¼ cup pepitas
½ cup sliced almonds

CANNED GOODS
2 cans (15 ounces each) full-fat coconut milk
1 can (15 ounces) Mexican stewed tomatoes
1 jar (16 ounces) mild green salsa
2 cans (15 ounces each) pinto beans
2 jars (8.5 ounces) sun-dried tomatoes, in oil
¼ cup tomato sauce
½ cup yellow Thai curry paste

GRAINS
2 cups brown rice
12 organic corn tortillas
5 cups quinoa, dry
2 cups red lentils, dry
2 cups white long grain rice

SEASONINGS
arrowroot powder
black pepper
chili powder
crushed red-pepper flakes
garlic powder
ground cumin
ground red pepper
Italian seasoning (or our Italian Herb Blend)
poppy seeds
sea salt

OPTIONAL
Italian Herb Blend
dried basil
dried oregano
dried marjoram
dried rosemary
dried thyme
dried parlsey
garlic powder
ground black pepper
red-pepper flakes

WEEK 2

DAY 1

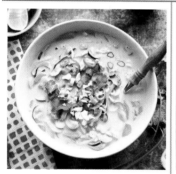

White Bean Soup, page 118

DAY 2

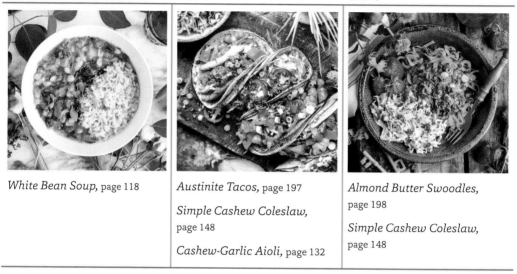

Austinite Tacos, page 197

Simple Cashew Coleslaw, page 148

Cashew-Garlic Aioli, page 132

DAY 3

Almond Butter Swoodles, page 198

Simple Cashew Coleslaw, page 148

DAY 4

Coconut Thai Soup, page 125

DAY 5

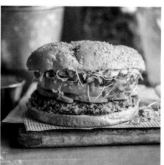

Garden Burgers, page 178

Baked Veggie Fries, page 171

Everything Bagel Sprinkle (optional), page 81

Homemade Ketchup (optional), page 171

shopping list

FRESH FRUIT
3 lemons
1 lime
1 avocado

FRESH VEGETABLES
1 cup baby bella mushrooms
7 carrots
1 head of cauliflower
2 ribs of celery
1 bunch of fresh cilantro
10 garlic cloves
1-inch ginger, fresh
2 cups green beans, fresh
½ head napa cabbage
1 bunch parsley, fresh
1 bunch scallions
1 serrano pepper
3 cups spinach
1 cup sprouts or microgreens
4 sweet potatoes
1 tomato
3 yellow onions
2 zucchini

OILS AND LIQUIDS
almond butter
apple cider vinegar
avocado oil
BBQ sauce
virgin coconut oil
Dijon mustard
tamari
6 cups vegetable stock
honey
maple syrup

NUTS AND SEEDS
1½ cups cashews, raw
½ cup sunflower seeds

CANNED GOODS
1 can (15 ounces) black beans
1 can (15 ounces) chickpeas
1 can (28 ounces) diced
  tomatoes
4 cans (13 ounces each)
  full-fat coconut milk
4 tablespoons red or green
  Thai curry paste
¼ cup sun-dried tomatoes,
  in oil
1 bag (16 ounces) cannellini
  beans, dry

GRAINS
2 cups brown rice
6 buns, whole wheat or
  gluten-free
12 organic corn tortillas
1 cup rolled oats, gluten-free

SEASONINGS
bay leaf
black pepper
chili powder
crushed red-pepper flakes
ground red pepper
oregano, dried
paprika
dried rosemary
sea salt
dried thyme
Italian Seasoning (or our
  Italian Herb Blend)
coconut sugar

OPTIONAL
Everything Bagel Sprinkle
dried minced garlic
dried minced onion
poppy seeds
sea salt
sesame seeds

Homemade Ketchup
apple cider vinegar
1 garlic clove
ground allspice
ground cinnamon
ground cloves
ground nutmeg
maple syrup
mustard powder
sea salt
1 can (6 ounces) tomato paste
½ cup tomato sauce
1 yellow onion

Italian Herb Blend
dried basil
dried oregano
dried marjoram
dried rosemary
dried thyme
dried parlsey
garlic powder
ground black pepper
red-pepper flakes

WEEK 3

DAY 1

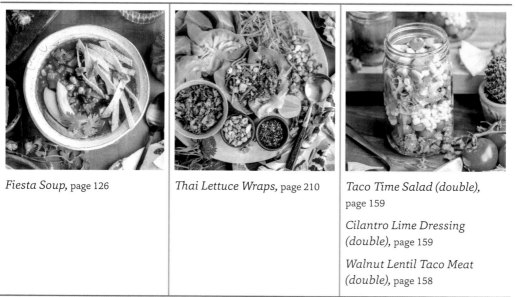

Fiesta Soup, page 126

DAY 2

Thai Lettuce Wraps, page 210

DAY 3

Taco Time Salad (double), page 159

Cilantro Lime Dressing (double), page 159

Walnut Lentil Taco Meat (double), page 158

DAY 4

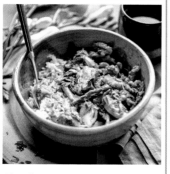

Simple Green Veggie Bowl, page 177

Blackened Sprouts, page 163

Coconut Sriracha Sauce, page 61

DAY 5

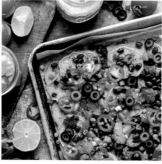

Plant-Powered Nachos (double), page 201

Spicy Avocado Crema, page 206

Cheeze Sprinkle, page 151

shopping list

FRESH FRUIT
11 limes
6 avocados

FRESH VEGETABLES
1 pound asparagus
8 ounces baby bella or white button mushrooms
1 pound Brussels sprouts
1 head of butter lettuce
2 carrots
1 rib of celery
2 cups cherry tomatoes
2 bunches of fresh cilantro
3 cups corn kernels, fresh or frozen
10 garlic cloves
fresh ginger
2 jalapeño peppers
1 bunch of fresh mint
1 red bell pepper
6 cups romaine lettuce
1 bunch of scallions
½ serrano pepper
1 shallot
4 sweet potatoes
2 tomatoes
1 yellow onion
1 zucchini

OILS AND LIQUIDS
almond butter
avocado oil
virgin coconut oil
Dijon mustard
extra-virgin olive oil
rice vinegar
Sriracha sauce
tamari
4 cups vegetable stock
honey
maple syrup

NUTS AND SEEDS
½ cup cashews, raw
4 cups walnuts

CANNED GOODS
2 cans (15 ounces) black beans
1 can (7 ounces) diced green chilies
1 can (15 ounces) diced tomatoes
¾ cup full-fat coconut milk
1 can (15 ounces) pinto beans
2 tablespoons tomato paste
1 cup sliced black olives

GRAINS
1½ cups brown rice
½ cup organic corn tortilla strips
1½ cups brown lentils

SEASONINGS
chili powder
cumin
garlic powder
nutritional yeast
paprika
crushed red-pepper flakes
sea salt
taco seasoning
coconut sugar

WEEK 4

DAY 1

Tex-Mex Breakfast Bowl,
page 67

Cashew Cream, page 67

Legit Salsa, page 91

DAY 2

Plant-Powered Cacao Chili,
page 182

*Almond Butter and Jam
Muffins,* page 76

*Strawberry Chia Jam
(optional),* page 75

DAY 3

Cauliflower Alfredo,
page 205

Italian Herb Blend (optional),
page 194

DAY 4

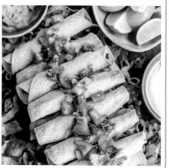

Black Bean Little Dippers,
page 181

Cashew Cream, page 67

Legit Salsa, page 91

Holy Guacamole, page 88

DAY 5

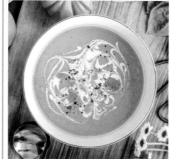

Sneaky Tomato Soup, page 123

shopping list

FRESH FRUIT
3 lemons
10 limes
7 avocados

FRESH VEGETABLES
1 bunch of fresh basil
2 bell peppers
1 cup broccoli florets
3 carrots
2 cups cauliflower florets
2 ribs of celery
1 bunch of fresh cilantro
1 cup corn kernels, frozen
18 garlic cloves
8 jalapeño peppers
1 poblano pepper
1 bunch of scallions
4 cups fresh spinach
1 tomato
6 yellow onions
3 zucchini

OILS AND LIQUIDS
almond milk, plain and
  unsweetened
apple cider vinegar
avocado oil
virgin coconut oil
Dijon mustard
honey
maple syrup
miso paste
4 cups vegetable stock
2 eggs

NUTS AND SEEDS
2 cup cashews, raw

CANNED GOODS
3 cans (15 ounces) black
  beans
1 can (28 ounces) crushed
  tomatoes
2 cans (28 ounces) diced
  tomatoes
1 can (15 ounces) kidney
  beans
1 can (15 ounces) pinto beans
½ cup sun-dried tomatoes

GRAINS
unbleached all-purpose flour
baking powder
1½ cups brown rice
24 6-inch organic corn
  tortillas
8 ounces gluten-free
  fettuccini
½ cup quinoa
3/4 cup stone-ground
  cornmeal

SEASONINGS
black pepper
cacao powder
chili powder
cinnamon
cumin
Italian seasoning (or our
  Italian Herb Blend)
nutmeg
nutritional yeast
crushed red-pepper flakes
sea salt

OPTIONAL
strawberry chia jam
chia seeds
fresh lemon juice
maple syrup
1 pound strawberries
pure vanilla extract

Italian Herb Blend
dried basil
dried oregano
dried marjoram
dried rosemary
dried thyme
dried parlsey
garlic powder
ground black pepper
red-pepper flakes

INDEX